'*Understanding Health, Illness and Society* is a lively, engagii introduction to health inequalities for undergraduate students. Through a rare combination of insight, humour, and academic rigor, Paton navigates the complexities between individual health and well-being and broader societal structures. This indispensable text should become the "go-to" for healthcare students and professionals seeking to understand sociology in health.'

Prof Kate Flemming PhD RN,
Department of Health Sciences, University of York, UK

'This book provides an excellent introduction to the relationship between health and society. The fact that it is written in an easily accessible and reader-friendly style commends it to every reader, but this book serves as a fantastic introduction for those healthcare students who have a desire to learn about the sociological aspects of healthcare (as all healthcare students should). I would certainly endorse this book to all pharmacy students.'

Dr Joseph Bush,
Dean of Aston Pharmacy School, Aston University, UK

'*Understanding Health, Illness and Society* is a wonderful book giving a valuable insight into to the social context of health and people's understanding of health. At a time when patient's needs are getting increasingly complex, it is important to understand the wider context of health. This book provides this context and more. Every doctor and medical student should read it.'

Dr Mumtaz Patel,
President, Royal College of Physicians, London, UK

Understanding Health, Illness and Society

This accessible book shows how social structures and social norms shape both individual and collective health. It provides readers with an insightful understanding of the relationship between society, health and illness and highlights issues to inform a progressive, patient-centred approach to contemporary healthcare.

The book begins by discussing how health has been defined and understood over the last century before examining how social issues such as deprivation, class, employment, housing, gender, ethnicity and policy shape health and contribute to health inequities. The book then discusses public health initiatives such as health promotion and screening programmes, the impact of resource allocation and the role that politics and policy play in supporting a healthy society. To bring concepts to life, the book uses case studies from the United Kingdom, the United States and Canada.

Guided by the fundamental principle that everything in a society has some effect or impact upon its health, and assuming no prior knowledge of the social sciences, this is the ideal book for healthcare students across nursing, medicine, midwifery and pharmacy, as well as anyone interested in the relationship between health and society.

Alexis Paton is Director of the Centre for Health and Society at Aston University, where she is a senior lecturer in social epidemiology and the sociology of health and the programme director of the Masters of Public Health. She is also the lead for the Social and Psychological Aspect of Health curriculum for Aston Medical School, where she has developed the current curriculum in line with General Medical Council requirements and learning outcomes for graduates.

Understanding Health, Illness and Society

A Patient-Centred Approach to Healthcare

Alexis Paton

Routledge
Taylor & Francis Group

LONDON AND NEW YORK

Designed cover image: Getty

First published 2026
by Routledge
4 Park Square, Milton Park, Abingdon, Oxon OX14 4RN

and by Routledge
605 Third Avenue, New York, NY 10158

Routledge is an imprint of the Taylor & Francis Group, an informa business

© 2026 Alexis Paton

British Library Cataloguing-in-Publication Data
A catalogue record for this book is available from the British Library

ISBN: 978-1-032-67756-9 (hbk)
ISBN: 978-1-032-67754-5 (pbk)
ISBN: 978-1-032-67755-2 (ebk)

DOI: 10.4324/9781032677552

Typeset in Sabon
by Apex CoVantage, LLC

This book is dedicated to two important people who have shaped my thinking. First, to the late Professor John A. Collins, my grandfather. A giant of obstetrics, reproductive medicine and evidence-based medicine, his life-long mentorship shaped my own drive to create an evidence base for health inequalities. It was in conversations with him that I developed my own professional views on why the determinants of health are so critical to good healthcare.

This book is also dedicated to my eldest daughter. Your curiosity for the world makes people think about why they hold beliefs and challenges them to change them, including me. Never stop being the kind, empathetic and questioning person that you are.

Contents

Acknowledgements

My immense thanks to Dee Cooke-Rees, without whom this book would be a sad and confused collection of unformatted gibberish. A thank you to Amy and Russell, who provided editorial support with the patience of saints and put up with more than a bit of stubbornness on my part.

To Steven, thank you for never losing faith, even when I did.

CHAPTER 1

Introduction

What is health?

Health is a complex thing: both subjective and objective. That which a person, society or profession understands to be healthy has never been fixed for long. In fact, some of what is taught now in medicine will have changed by the time you consider yourself a senior member of a health profession. This is an inevitability of the forward march of science but also, crucially for the subject of this book, a defining feature of the continual shifting sands of cultural and societal change. Within our own lives, our own definitions that we hold for our own individual health—our own idea of 'healthy'—will change with our circumstances: ageing, parenthood (or not), injury, employment. All these seemingly unscientific, unmedical phenomena—the collection of things that make up our lives—will profoundly influence what we ourselves consider to be a healthy life.

The concept of health is so changeable that it can often come as a surprise to those entering or already in the health professions. While presented largely as a scientific pursuit in school, medicine is not black and white; it is less concrete and absolute in practice than it is so often portrayed. It has trends, gaps in its knowledge and areas of deliberate 'unknowing' due to the largely unscientific influences on what is considered important in health and medicine itself. Health is never perfect; nor is medicine. Both are influenced by the world around us, and thus both its and our own understandings of health never stand still for very long.

In this book, we will examine the ever-changing world of health by looking at the phenomena (things that happen around us that we can experience and feel) that impact on individual health, societal understanding of health and public health more widely. Our focus will chiefly be the way the world in which we live influences and acts on our health, showing 'health' for the precarious concept that it is. My hope is that in understanding the many different ways that health is shaped by simple things, such as what we eat, where we live or how much money we make, it will help you to understand, support and treat your patients better in your daily practice. When someone comes to you in ill health, the story behind it will often be much more complicated than a virus, an injury or a collection of symptoms. If you can understand the complexity of health,

DOI: 10.4324/9781032677552-1

the messiness of human life that shapes health, then you will have a fighting chance of promoting, supporting and even restoring 'good' health (whatever 'good health' means in that moment).

To help with this, we will cover a variety of (often) seemingly 'un-health' concepts—but stay with me, as each of these is vital for understanding health in your professional life. I will even be so bold as to say that understanding these concepts will likely make you a better healthcare professional, full stop. We will begin with a brief history of health and medicine in order to understand the changes in definitions of health and how they have culminated in our current, globally accepted WHO definition of health. We will then move on to look more specifically at the context of health: what are known as the social and structural determinants (meaning influences) of health and how they shape our own beliefs and behaviours around health in turn. We will also look at the way understandings and beliefs about health translate into medical practice at both the individual and population levels. Of course, most aspects of society are well beyond our control and so we will also spend some time unpacking the impact of politics, policy and cultural trends on health. Finally, I hope to give you some food for thought on the future of medicine and how it must meet the problem of climate change head-on and rise to the challenge of sustainability to keep populations healthy for generations to come.

However, before we discuss what health is or even what health should be, let us go back a bit to understand what health has meant over the past few centuries in the Euro-American context. As we do, I want you to remember that across the globe, there are many different ways of understanding health. I focus on the Euro-American context because that is the one I know the best and the one that many of you will work in one day. It is not a judgement on a 'right' or 'wrong' way of understanding health and medicine. It is instead a continents-wide case study of the strength of the influence of the social world on health and medicine. Were we to undertake this same exercise in another part of the world, this chapter, and indeed large parts of this book, would look very different. In fact, others have done so, and I encourage you to read about health and medicine worldwide as part of your life-long learning in the field.

A brief history of health and medicine (mostly in Europe)
Go back about 800 years to medieval Europe and you would see that much like today, health was most often about access to food, water and shelter. Without these three, good health is easily lost and poor health sets in. Living conditions were, as they are now, paramount to living a healthy life. Oddly, much of what was the norm out of necessity in previous centuries is now a coveted part of a healthy lifestyle. Home-grown fruit and vegetables were the main part of most diets. All food was effectively organic, with few pollutants in the waterways and wells (if you don't count animal and human excrement). Daily exercise was a common and necessary part of life.

Before you get overly nostalgic, there were, of course, some rather notable drawbacks. Living in cramped quarters meant that waste was often not disposed of in ways that prevented infection and disease. Harvests dictated what was available to eat and storage of food was limited. Most people shared their home at night with farm animals and small houses were constantly choked by soot from open fires. Women never knew if their next baby would be the literal death of them. Arguably, a happier, healthier time it was most likely not.

So why have I taken you down this rather grim memory lane? Because looking to the past in this way helps to build a picture of health as a relatively simple thing that can be wildly thrown off course by the world that we live in. Medieval Europe is a stark, yet excellent, example of just how strong an influence the social world has on our health. Take medicine at that time: for nearly 300 years, science, which was a very fluid concept indeed back then, had little to do with health in the minds of the continent's inhabitants. Religion, in the form of Christianity, was the absolute cornerstone of European society and culture. As a result, religion played a huge part in medicine for several hundred years. With limited understanding of germ theory and infection pathways, illness and disease were viewed as punishments from God or a test of faith. Some even welcomed ill health as a way to show their devotion to God. Medicine from that time would be unrecognisable to us today, but to the average medieval person, pneumonia as punishment for, say, taking the Lord's name in vain, seemed fair and explainable. It made sense within the culture of the time and was accepted as truth.

In those times, if someone was ill, they might have their cold diagnosed via a study of the stars and their treatment might be a religious charm given to them by a monk or nun. There was no professionalisation of medicine; it was not the career we know today. There was no governance or certification for most individuals who practised medicine. 'Barber surgeons' operated unchecked, though they had usually apprenticed in some way with older surgeons. Wise women and apothecaries were the community sources of care. Those who were very rich and lucky would attend one of those new-fangled 'universities' to become a physician. You might be interested to know that the degree took about as long as it does now, but students spent most of it reading ancient Greek texts about astrology and learning to diagnose without ever touching a patient. A full star chart was needed to work out under which Zodiac sign and planet an ailment had appeared, before an equally complex remedy, harvested and prepared under the correct night sky, was administered. Sounds like a pain in the butt? Don't worry, those normally show up when the moon appears in Virgo. You'll need an infusion made from henbane plucked when Mars is in retrograde.

No, seriously. How humans survived to this point almost defies the laws of evolution. It's safe to say that there were a few gaps in knowledge even among medieval boffins. Frankly, I'd rather have taken my chances with the wise women and barber surgeons—they at least received hands-on clinical training.

What is interesting about medieval health and medicine is that it took the concept of wealth equals good health, a concept that we will discuss at length in this book, to the very extreme. Money could (and still does) buy people better food, more meat and fish, better grain, sturdier and bigger homes, a barn for their animals so they didn't have to bunk with cows every night—even drainage and a better water supply could be bought if they had the cash. Indeed, medieval Europe, out of the entire history of medicine, is the perfect example of why it matters so much for our health that we understand the world within which medicine is practised. The influence of the social world on health in history is stark. It shows us how a bad harvest, a good day at market or an overcrowded house could mean the difference between a healthy life and an unhealthy life. The fact that those things STILL mean the difference between good and ill health should show you how important the social world is to health and medicine.

Back then, societal beliefs around health meant that health was an individual affair. People lived and died by their good health, which was largely their own responsibility. The chest infection they could not shake—they had brought that on themself and must bear the burden of it. There was no concept of the government playing any part in health and medicine. Those who could afford a doctor paid for one, and those who could not, took their chances in monasteries and convents or were simply cared for and died at home. Shocked? Don't be. In parts of the world, this is largely still both the ideology around health (that it is our own personal responsibility) and the pay-at-point-of-access healthcare that many countries have adopted. Neither concept sprang from nowhere; in fact the roots go extremely deep.

Luckily for Europe and Britain, there was a shift in cultural and societal beliefs around health and medicine in the late nineteenth century that would shape our modern understanding of both. All of a sudden, caring about others became important and the government was expected to get involved. Health became of interest to the nation and as such, the responsibility for good health was seen, at least in part, as that of the government. This brought the professionalisation of medicine and public health to the scene.

Medicine in the nineteenth century

By the time of the industrial revolution, Britain was a different place. Urban centres were crowded and new advances in technology meant that new social classes were emerging within society. Globally, science was changing too. Microscopes, for example, allowed for an exploration of a minute world in plain sight. The discovery of germ theory by Pasteur, showing that bacteria were a cause of disease, took hold, changing the scientific and, ultimately, the cultural understanding of who was to blame for ill health. With the influence of religion waning, Britain, like other countries, was beginning to see that illness was more complex. God could not be argued with, but if it were bacteria that actually spread disease, then things like the spread of cholera could be controlled. Infection control measures meant that illness was not out of our hands—it was literally in our hands, as hand-washing, sterilisation, pasteurisation and vaccines meant that good health was becoming more widely obtainable and medicine had an important role to play in maintaining it. This shift in understanding the responsibility of health and the cause of disease shows the importance of beliefs about good and ill health in the way we treat health. If a person is not responsible for bringing illness upon themself, then they should be supported in getting treatment for that illness: someone has to take responsibility. Thus, the professionalisation of medicine began; because if someone needed to take responsibility, then there needed to be rules and regulations around who could be a doctor, what being a doctor meant and what was expected of those who are doctors. For you doctors reading this, remember that the next time you pay the General Medical Council (GMC) your annual fees, it's really Pasteur's fault that you have to pay anything in the first place.

The nineteenth century, thus, ushered in not just a new understanding of health but also of healthcare too. We will see this as a theme again and again: beliefs around health influence policy, practice and healthcare, as well as the other way around.

Medicine is not developed or practised in a vacuum but right in the messy thick of the social world.

Being a professional means not just having status and authority over the subject of that profession but also a responsibility to self-regulate, control and organise the profession. Professions are characterised by an autonomy—an ability to decide what counts as the profession, who can join (and who can't, which is equally important), how people learn the profession and the ethics (the dos and don'ts of the profession). Medicine is no different. The 1858 Medical Act established a legal and societal obligation to self-regulate and instituted what we know today as the GMC, the regulatory body of medicine in the United Kingdom (Waddington, 1990). The Act gave the GMC the power and responsibility to regulate medicine as a profession, including the provision of medical education and maintaining a register of qualified doctors. In many ways its role is very similar today. Interestingly, at that time, people could still practise medicine unqualified, but they would not be allowed to do so for any government services. Much like today, they could engage in any quackery or snake oil selling that they wanted, but not on the government's dime—the authorities would not contract people or pay them to care for others if they were unqualified. However, people could take that risk themselves if they wanted to, and they still do today. We will talk about that a few chapters from now.

However, professionalisation eventually does push out the unqualified, especially if it is the only way to make any money from the profession. In the late nineteenth century, registration with the GMC rapidly became the goal for those who wanted to become or were doctors. To do so, doctors needed to meet their ever-increasing standards of education, eventually resulting in the governance body that we recognise today as the GMC. In fact, the GMC developed such high standards regarding who could practise (including education and ethics) that, by the 1880s, there were so few qualified doctors that a workforce shortage loomed (Waddington, 1990). If this sounds familiar, know that the take-home message of much of this book is that, eventually, everything old is new again.

While the professionalisation of medicine can be seen as an important and much-needed step forward in establishing the safe and effective medicine we recognise today, it was also a chance for exclusion based on the prevailing societal beliefs of the day. Nineteenth-century medicine and the regulatory bodies that governed it were, in the Anglo-American and European worlds at least, a product of the racist and misogynistic culture of the time (Remedium, 2022; Daher et al., 2021; Jarral, 2016). It was rare for someone from an ethnic minority background to attend the medical schools that were being codified and officially recognised in the nineteenth century. Dr James McCune Smith, the first Black man to be awarded a medical degree in the United Kingdom at the University of Glasgow, may have had the paperwork to practise—but he was denied entry to most medical associations at the time, including the American Medical Association in the United States (Morgan, 2003, p. 7), where he lived and worked. The fact that Smith spent his entire career not only treating patients as a doctor but also methodically and scientifically refuting the racist bunk about the inferiority of 'non-white' people in his native United States speaks volumes to his intelligence and commitment to improving medical practice in his own era. Though there are few historical accounts of Smith, the existing evidence indicates that he was interested in understanding and helping those who society would prefer to ignore and even forget.

Unsurprisingly, he was a supporter of the suffragette movement and held evening classes in his own house to teach reading, writing and arithmetic (Morgan, 2003, p. 7). He was a pioneer of infection control, insisting on administering the smallpox vaccine to the children in the orphanage where he worked and advocating to control overcrowding and improve ventilation (Morgan, 2003, p. 7). With opium having been a more popular drug of choice at that time, he was also interested in the relationship between opium, menstruation and the possibility of it helping in menopause—two topics of conversation that never saw the light of day back then (or, some may argue, even now, but that's for another chapter). I could go on, and other historians have, but I hope this gives an idea of how much can be lost from the practice of medicine due to simple and prejudiced beliefs about who is worthy to practise a profession when that profession is officially recognised and governed by those in a position of oppressive power. The history of medicine is one of white, male supremacy, and we cannot forget this when we look at the influence that the social world has had on health and medicine.

Women have suffered a similar fate in the history of health and medicine. Since Henry VIII's (that great champion of women . . . I hope my disdain is evident here) 1540 charter that formed the Company of Barber Surgeons, women were specifically excluded from the professional world of medicine. This persisted for well over 300 years. Misogynistic viewpoints saw women as incapable of dealing with the gory mess that medicine can be (Jarral, 2016)—an odd stance, given the monthly gore of menstruation and the clinical skill required for successful childbirth, but then it perhaps goes without saying that gynaecology lagged behind as a speciality of medicine for several centuries, packaged as 'women's troubles' that were best left alone. Women in Britain had to set up their own schools and hospitals; the British Medical Association did not admit them until 1892 (Lamont, 1992) and only because female doctors battled for that recognition. Professionalisation has a dark side, keeping out those whom the society has judged unworthy to practise medicine, rather than accounting for ability.

This exclusion, based on cultural beliefs in society, has had clinical consequences that we still feel in medicine today. Women's health has in general been less well researched and poorly understood, and as a result it is still harder to diagnose and treat (Criado Pérez, 2019). For anyone who isn't white, medicine is even further behind; many medical textbooks still only feature white subjects (Mukwende et al., 2020) and continue to under-educate on very simple and life-saving clinical differences, such as rash presentation on darker skin. The beliefs resulting from 800 years of prejudice still haunt modern medicine today.

Health and medicine in the twentieth and twenty-first centuries

Fast forward to the 1900s and things started to change. Alongside professionalisation, despite a 'plus ca change' stagnation in cultural beliefs, what health was—how it was defined and understood—was changing too. Health had been both a basic thing (food, water, shelter) and a complex thing (wrath of God, crossed star signs and 'foul air') for several hundred years, but it was now understood to be wholly discoverable and understandable through science. The biomedical model of health was born.

Perhaps the most pervasive (and some argue the most damaging) way of understanding health, the biomedical model of health dominated medicine for well over a hundred years. With religion and mysticism banished from Euro-American concepts of health and medicine, the biomedical model celebrated the revolutionary medical science that characterised health and healthcare from the twentieth century onwards.

So what is it—this seemingly amazing concept that is the foundation of modern medicine today?

As healthcare students, you're probably in your programme because you want to learn about how the body works: how it can go wrong and how to fix it. Under the biomedical model, 'the body is treated like a machine that is fixed by removing or replacing the ailing part or destroying the foreign body that is causing the problem' (McClelland, 1985). Essentially, your patient is a car with a dodgy engine noise and you are the mechanic sent in to sort it. I know. Even as I write this analogy, I can hear your outrage. People are not just a collection of parts—but for about a hundred years, during which many of your parents and even my ageing self were born, that was the dominant understanding of health in medicine. As a result, health was understood as an absence of disease (Hart, 1985). The doctor's role was to make that disease disappear and maintain health for the patient.

Twentieth-century medicine was characterised by doctors working to make disease absent—focusing on anatomy, physiology and the biological causes of disease in order to make people healthy and keep them that way (Hart, 1985). Medicine, then, was not really interested in things like psychological problems, health behaviours or people's social context. These were understood as outside of the remit of doctors—nothing to do with them. Mental wellbeing was not medicine. The mind was not a machine.

The biomedical model comes from dualist philosophy (I know, its humanities, but stay with me here). Dualism views the mind and body as separate and independent entities. The body is seen as having material properties and obeying the laws of physics, essentially working like a machine, whereas the mind is viewed as free of all that (Calef, n.d.). The mind is an unencumbered, disembodied, non-physical substance that dualists are very sure is not a brain, and yet whenever I try to reconcile dualism with the real world, I only see brains floating in vats, like in those weird mobile phone adverts for VOXI in 2023.

This focus has obviously been associated with major advances in modern medicine. It has led to huge improvements in the understanding of disease and major advances in treatment, from the development of vaccines to the whole armoury of drugs and surgical procedures available to patients today. I'd be lying if I said that the era of the biomedical model is over. It does continue to be prominent in modern medicine, and for some people in ill health, it makes logical sense to think in this way. But people are more than just the sum of their parts. In the language of the biomedical model, we are part machine, yes, but in a sort of cuddly cyborg way. We are Robocop, wrestling with our humanity, while also understanding the usefulness of antibiotics to see off sepsis. So, what is the alternative?

The biopsychosocial model of health

The biomedical model has been criticised as far too narrow an approach to understanding health and illness because it ignores the influence of social and psychological factors on health. We are our bodies (bio), our minds (psycho) and our world (social) around us, and so our understanding of health must reflect this mix. By the mid-twentieth century, The World Health Organisation (WHO) was critical of the biomedical model, and so in 1948, it released its own definition of health as part of its constitution, one that it still holds today:

> Health is a state of complete physical, mental and social well-being and not merely the absence of disease or infirmity.
>
> *(World Health Organisation, 1948).*

This was a bold and strong statement from the WHO; it sent the message that all three of these aspects of human life must be attended to and considered when supporting a person's health. Over the next 30 years or so, the dominance of the biomedical model of health was no longer sitting well with many practising clinicians. A population that had withstood two world wars (and more to come) was understandably having some difficulty processing things. Clear links could be drawn between mental wellbeing, health and the social world. In 1977, George Engel, an American psychiatrist, came up with a new way of describing the holistic vision he had for practising medicine and understanding health: the biopsychosocial model of health (Engel, 1977) (Figure 1.1).

The biopsychosocial model of health struck an immediate chord; it remains the ethos of Euro-American medicine to this day. The model describes health and illness as complex and emerging from an interplay of biological, social and psychological factors. The 'BIO' factors refer to what we know and continue to learn from the science of health and medicine: things such as human physiology, genetics and pathogens. The 'PSYCHO' factors refer to the way people think, feel and behave. It recognises mental wellbeing, cognition and emotion as a critical part of health. Finally, the 'SOCIAL'

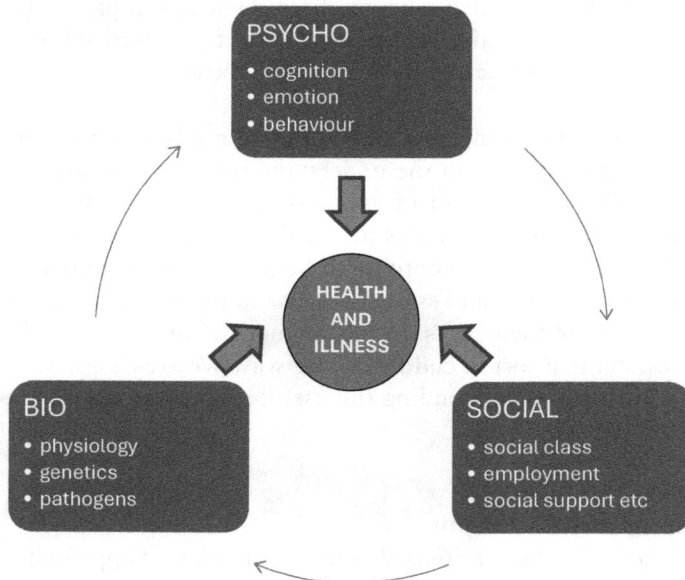

Figure 1.1 The Biopsychosocial Model of Health.

factors refer to a wide range of issues relating to the world in which people live and embody their own health. It includes all the seemingly 'non-health' aspects that influence and shape health, including socio-economic status, housing and employment, social support, gender and ethnicity. Engel argued that each of these feed into our own health; in particular, we need to look beyond the biology of health and understand that psychological and social factors are contributing causes of illness and that medicine needs to take this complex picture into account, both for preventing and treating disease. However, health is not all individual; sometimes it takes a village to keep that village healthy.

Public versus individual health

While various conceptions of health were developing, one aspect grew steadily: the idea of public health. With the abandonment of the personal responsibility approach to health in the nineteenth century, the rise of public health—the idea that a country must care for and promote good health in its population—was a logical next step. Britain didn't always get this right, so let us take a brief foray into the history of public health in Britain to understand better how we conceptualise health.

When Henry VIII was having a massive strop over his own infertility, he dissolved the religious houses that had been among the few places ordinary people could access healthcare and support. To try and restore a way to support those in need, the Poor Relief Act became law in 1601. It was a very simple form of the national insurance and council support we know today. Local parishes collected taxes, which in turn were used to support people who could not work (UK Parliament, 2015). Like so many acts of parliament, it was no silver bullet. Societal ideas about who was to blame for ill health had a heavy influence. Prevailing ideas about individual responsibility for health were still strong—so much so that in 1834 the Poor Relief Act morphed into the monstrous Poor Law Amendment that saw the opening of workhouses. Workhouses were hideous, dystopian-style institutions where poor people, including children, were forced to work as indentured servants in exchange for (minimal) food, clothing and shelter. It was the 'hostile environment' of its time, with the instigator, Edwin Chadwick (incidentally a man who had clearly never fallen on hard times in his life—otherwise why would he create such a thing?), arguing that if the solution to poverty was made unpleasant, people would be motivated not to be poor and poverty would cease to exist (UK Parliament, n.d.a). If only the solution were that simple, Edwin. It certainly was unpleasant, so he succeeded in that at least. Credit where credit is due and all that.

At some point Chadwick seems to have had a (slight) change of heart, changing tack and arguing that actually if we could keep the poor healthy, the economy would be much healthier too. In that, he was not wrong, but he and I have very different ideas about what constitutes 'keeping the poor healthy', so that is about as much as I am willing to give him. The 1848 Public Health Act established a Central Board of Health and provided a framework for local authorities to use. The idea was that they would use loans from the government to provide and improve key aspects of good health at the time: clean water supplies, drainage and infrastructure changes such as paving roads. Even the UK Parliament recognises that it was not a perfect system. The act gave the central board and local authorities very little power to enforce change, but it was a step in the right direction (UK Parliament, n.d.a), and, crucially, it passed the responsibility for promoting good health to the government.

By 1942, more compassionate minds had seen sense, and the Beveridge Report criticised the Poor Law as the grotesque, out-of-date beast that it was, arguing for a welfare state that would care for British citizens 'from cradle to grave' (UK Parliament, n.d.b). The idea of a welfare state made room in the social and political beliefs of the time for what the United Kingdom now calls its National Health Service (NHS), established in 1948. Whatever health was, it was no longer the individual's sole responsibility. The state, in this case the British government, was considered to play an important role in supporting and maintaining people's health.

Once again, the definition of health had shifted. Wealth was not the only means by which to access health and healthcare. Free at the point of use, the NHS in Britain represented a change in the social and cultural understandings of health that continue to shape how health is viewed in Britain today. Political movements and Conservative and Labour governments have come and gone, yet the idea that Britain must provide free healthcare to its citizens has thus far remained a quintessential part of 'being British'.

Most European countries have similar stories. Universal healthcare, meaning free (or very close to free) access to healthcare, is the norm throughout Europe. Out of the wider Euro-American medical tradition we've been covering in this chapter, only the United States operates outside of a broadly universal healthcare system, continuing to view (at least in policy, if not in wider ethos) health as a personal responsibility, with individuals bearing the costs for their own health. This is unsurprising given the history of the United States; it is the birthplace of libertarianism, an ideology that values autonomy and the ability for someone to make their own choices about themself—and no one else—above all else (van der Vossen and Christmas, 2024). Taken in the context of health, this means a person is not responsible for someone else's health, only their own. Universal healthcare systems most often use taxes or some version of national insurance to cover the costs of healthcare. In the libertarian world, this is considered taking away one person's hard-earned money to give to someone else. Brutal, but a fundamental concept in one of the world's most powerful countries, and a very good example of how strongly a societal belief about health can shape not just an individual's health but that of a whole country. The fact that whole lives have been destroyed by a single hospital bill has done nothing to change the system in the United States; rather shockingly, most US doctors remain in favour of the pay-for-use system they work in. In fact, the American Medical Association ran a campaign against the introduction of Medicare, the system for accessible healthcare for the elderly, in the hopes of destroying what they considered to be the introduction of a 'socialist' medical system (Altom and Churchill, 2007). The beliefs of a society, culture or country are instrumental in the way they understand health, shaping their policies and practices around healthcare.

Medicine and health in the twenty-first century
So here we are, about a quarter of the way through the twenty-first century, and I bet you are wondering what we think about health now. Maybe even thinking: how do those beliefs about health shape the way we practise medicine? If you are, I'm proud of you. We will get along fine in this book. Health in the twenty-first century is as complex as ever. For the past 20-odd years, in the face of economic recession and

political instability, the idea of health as a personal responsibility has begun to gain ground again. Remember, everything old is so often new again when it comes to health. While health as a personal responsibility was more of a *laissez-faire*, the government-does-not-intervene-in-personal-lives concept prior to the nineteenth century, personal responsibility for health is now more about blame and controlling who can access healthcare.

Britain has been at the forefront of this trend for some time, especially with regards to obesity. Being overweight is so strongly linked to the idea of personal responsibility for health that it is a common belief that overweight people bring their health problems upon themselves. Personal responsibility is a key part of the political, cultural, social and even legal approaches that countries and healthcare systems take when trying to reduce obesity in their populations (Brownell et al., 2010). The language used is purposeful—it is designed to make people think that fat people are lazy, weak, prone to vice and excess and thus directly responsible for their own ill health. The point is to create a belief that weight is ONLY controlled by the individual who bears it. This allows for a passing of the buck, a stepping back from governments around obesity that ignores many of the key causes of obesity to begin with—causes that are, as you can guess, largely societal and cultural, with some genetics thrown in too. In short, things that are mostly out of people's individual control (Paton, 2020; Sim, 2017).

The result of this 'responsibilisation' of health, as seen through the case study of obesity, is that we practise medicine differently. In the case of obesity, many treatments for disease unrelated to obesity, for example infertility, require individuals to lose weight before they will allow them to be eligible for the treatment. There are, of course, some instances where weight loss is helpful, for example in the recovery from certain surgeries. But while there are some (mildly) elevated risks to a fat pregnancy, it hardly seems a fair reason to deny someone the chance to have a child by requiring a certain BMI for fertility treatment—especially when weight has nothing to do with one's ability to parent. We discuss in detail why social determinants are such a huge factor in things like obesity further on in the book. My goal right now is to help you understand, again, that what we believe in our social lives, in the culture where we live, shapes the way we understand health to such an extent that it can change our health too because it changes our access to healthcare.

Epigenetics—is it all relative? Or at least contextual?
Before we dive into the social determinants of health in our next chapter, I want to leave you with one final thought on what health is now. As I said above, health is currently viewed simultaneously as our responsibility and not our responsibility, depending on who you ask. We are divided in our understanding of what constitutes health and a healthy life. But do we have any control at all? It's worth considering this question when thinking about the growing trend of understanding health through the lens of epigenetics and personalised medicine. Again, as with our scientific buddies from the 1800s, leaps ahead in science are shedding new light on our understandings of health and illness.

I know I've ragged on the biomedical model A LOT in this chapter, so you can be forgiven if you've either forgotten about the 'bio' part of medicine, or, much more likely, been screaming at me for the last several thousand words that it is important. It is important. I agree. We are, after all, biological creatures, animals developed through time and evolution to the humans we are today. We are who we are due in large part to our genes. This is where we find the fascinating world of epigenetics and a glimpse into the way twenty-first century medicine may be remembered by history.

Genes play an important role in health. They are the blueprint for the building blocks of life, proteins. DNA is the factory manual for our body, with genes being read and proteins being produced constantly. In theory, in a stable vacuum, that DNA would be read effectively the same way every time. Mutations would occur—don't get me wrong, they are an inevitability of the whole DNA process—but the reading and expressing of genes would stay the same. However, humans do not live in a stable vacuum. We live complex, messy lives, subject to forces and environments often largely outside of our control. These forces are not banal. Just as society shapes our beliefs about health, the environment we live in and even some of our behaviours can shape and change how our bodies read the blueprint of our DNA (US Centers for Disease Control and Prevention, n.d.).

This is epigenetics: the way that outside environmental influences change how our genes are read and expressed. Unlike mutations, these changes are not irreversible—in fact, they often change as we age. The epigenome is a collection of chemical markers that affect how a gene is read. Different experiences influence the epigenome, shifting it about and dictating exactly how much, if any, of a gene can be expressed at any given time (Harvard University Center on the Developing Child, 2019). These influences can be positive (i.e. opportunities for learning, a safe home environment and suffi-cient nutrition) or negative (a stressful home life or exposure to environmental toxins). Children, in particular, are susceptible to these changes, which can have long-lasting influences on abilities such as learning or even how tall they grow or how much they weigh.

Epigenetics may be one way of developing a more personalised medicine. Personalised medicine based on our own unique genome is considered a potential way forward for combatting disease (European Commission, n.d.). In many ways it makes sense. Many people have preferences for over-the-counter medication, believing that ibuprofen is more effective than paracetamol, for example, and for them it may very well be. We are all unique and these differences show up in both our susceptibility to disease and our acceptance and tolerance of the treatments for those diseases. If we can develop an indi-vidual cheat sheet of what might work most effectively for each person—and further personalise that by harnessing epigenetics to express the right amount of gene at the right time—then for once 'personal responsibility' in medicine might actually be a posi-tive thing. New forays into genetic medicine, including the editing of faulty genes, have already begun, with cautiously optimistic outcomes (Bowen-Metcalf, 2023). Again, the way we define health is changing. It may be possible to build a healthier person in the future, but before we do, we should ask ourselves: do we want to?

Conclusion

What will all these changes mean for health and the way we understand what health is? We at least have to ask the question. Will it change the way we understand health to know exactly how much of our good and ill health is, in many ways, pre-ordained through our genes? Are we back to the biomedical model in some ways? Are we just a pile of DNA strands, twisting in the metaphorical wind? What happens to our understanding of health when we inevitably come up against diseases that we cannot 'fix' with genetics? It may all feel a bit sci-fi, but the possibility that personalised medicine creates a stratification of healthier and unhealthier social groups that is even more stark than the one we currently have is something we have to think about now, when we have the chance to ensure that this doesn't happen as a result of the forward march in medical progress.

I hope that this chapter has shown you that so much of health and medicine is swept up in the tsunami of scientific discovery and the prevailing social beliefs of the day. With epigenetics and personalised medicine there is a possible moment of pause to work out how to practise medicine and understand health in a way that does not further disenfranchise sections of our population. It is not my intention to throw you into an existential crisis before you even finish the first chapter of this book, but it is worth considering how jarring the idea is that health is our own personal responsibility when the world we live in literally changes how our genes are expressed, thus changing who we are. There are very few ways that we can control these changes, but it is possible. As we will see throughout the rest of this book, where we live, what we do for a job, how much money we have, what we eat and how we learn are critical to our understanding of health and to the extent to which we can actually be healthy. Epigenetics and the social world are both places where what someone has and who they are can make the difference between a healthy life and an unhealthy one. Health is not all relative. However, like so much in life, it is contextual, and that is the focus of this book: to show how the societal and cultural contexts of our lives weave together to create good or ill health.

References

Altom, L.K. and Churchill, L.R. (2007). 'Pay, pride, and public purpose: Why America's doctors should support universal healthcare.' *Medscape General Medicine* 9(1): 40. Available at: https://www.ncbi.nlm.nih.gov/pmc/articles/PMC1925024/

Bowen-Metcalf, G. (2023). 'What is gene editing and how could it shape our future?' *The Conversation*, 14th February. Available at: https://theconversation.com/what-is-gene-editing-and-how-could-it-shape-our-future-199025

Brownell, K.D., Kersh, R., Ludwig, D.S., Post, R.C., Puhl, R.M., Schwartz, M.B. and Willett, W.C. (2010). 'Personal responsibility and obesity: A constructive approach to a controversial issue.' *Health Affairs (Millwood)* 29(3): 379–387. https://doi.org/10.1377/hlthaff.2009.0739.

Calef, S. (n.d.). 'Dualism and mind.' *Internet Encyclopedia of Philosophy*. Available at: https://iep.utm.edu/dualism-and-mind

Criado Pérez, C. (2019). *Invisible women*. London: Chatto & Windus.

Daher, Y., Austin, E.T., Munter, B.T., Murphy, L. and Gray, K. (2021). 'The history of medical education: A commentary on race.' *Journal of Osteopathic Medicine* 121(2): 163–170. https://doi.org/10.1515/jom-2020-0212

Engel, G.L. (1977). 'The need for a new medical model: A challenge for biomedicine.' *Science* 196(4286): 129–136. Available at: https://www.science.org/doi/10.1126/science.847460

European Commission (n.d.). *Personalised medicine*. Available at: https://health.ec.europa.eu/medicinal-products/personalised-medicine_en

Hart, N. (1985). *The sociology of health and medicine*. Lancashire: Causeway Press.

Harvard University Center on the Developing Child (2019). *Epigenetics and child development: How children's experiences affect their genes*. Available at: https://developingchild.harvard.edu/resources/what-is-epigenetics-and-how-does-it-relate-to-child-development/

Jarral, F. (2016). 'No scrubs: How women had to fight to become doctors.' *The Guardian*, 26th September. Available at: https://www.theguardian.com/lifeandstyle/2016/sep/26/no-scrubs-how-women-had-to-fight-to-become-doctors

Lamont, T. (1992). 'The Amazons within: Women in the BMA 100 years ago.' *British Medical Journal* 305: 1529–1532. Available at: https://www.ncbi.nlm.nih.gov/pmc/articles/PMC1884708/pdf/bmj00105-0021.pdf

McClelland, D.C. (1985). 'The social mandate of health psychology.' *American Behavioral Scientist* 28(4): 451–467. https://doi.org/10.1177/000276485028004003

Morgan, T.M. (2003). 'The education and medical practice of Dr. James McCune Smith (1813–1865), first black American to hold a medical degree.' *Journal of the National Medical Association* 95(7) (July): 603–614. Available at: https://www.ncbi.nlm.nih.gov/pmc/articles/PMC2594637

Mukwende, M., Tamony, P. and Turner, M. (2020). *Mind the gap: A handbook of clinical signs in Black and Brown skin*. London: St George's, University of London. Available at: https://www.blackandbrownskin.co.uk/mindthegap

Paton, A. (2020). 'I'm worried about Boris Johnson's plan to tackle obesity—the government cannot abandon its responsibility to the public.' *The Independent*, 22nd July. Available at: https://www.independent.co.uk/voices/boris-johnson-obesity-coronavirus-nhs-healthcare-a9632881.html

Remedium (2022). *Black history month: The history of Black healthcare professionals in the NHS*. Available at: https://remediumpartners.com/black-history-month-the-history-of-black-healthcare-professionals-in-the-nhs

Sim, F. (2017). 'Obesity—personal responsibility or environmental curse?' *The BMJ Opinion*, 24th October. Available at: https://blogs.bmj.com/bmj/2017/10/24/fiona-sim-obesity-personal-responsibility-or-environmental-curse/

UK Parliament (2015). *1601 poor law*. Available at: https://www.parliament.uk/about/living-heritage/evolutionofparliament/2015-parliament-in-the-making/get-involved1/2015-banners-exhibition/rachel-gadsden/1601-poor-law-gallery

UK Parliament (n.d.a). *The 1848 public health act*. Available at: https://www.parliament.uk/about/living-heritage/transformingsociety/towncountry/towns/tyne-and-wear-case-study/about-the-group/public-administration/the-1848-public-health-act/ [accessed 7th August 2024].

UK Parliament (n.d.b). *1942 Beveridge report*. Available at: https://www.parliament.uk/about/living-heritage/transformingsociety/livinglearning/coll-9-health1/coll-9-health/

US Centers for Disease Control and Prevention (n.d.). *Epigenetics, health, and disease*. Available at: https://www.cdc.gov/genomics-and-health/about/epigenetic-impacts-on-health.html

van der Vossen, B. and Christmas, B. (2024). 'Libertarianism.' In *The Stanford encyclopedia of philosophy* [Winter 2024 Edition], edited by E.N. Zalta and U. Nodelman. Available at: https://plato.stanford.edu/archives/win2024/entries/libertarianism

Waddington, I. (1990). 'The movement towards the professionalisation of medicine.' *British Medical Journal* 301: 688–90. Available at: https://www.ncbi.nlm.nih.gov/pmc/articles/PMC1664090/pdf/bmj00199-0018.pdf

World Health Organisation (1948). *Constitution*. Available at: https://www.who.int/about/governance/constitution

The social context of health

The social and structural determinants of health

When we think about health, it is mostly good news. We are living longer and more healthily than we have in a long time. Over the last 40 years or so, our life expectancy has been slowly increasing thanks to advances in medicine and social care (Office for National Statistics, 2024). There is, in Britain and much of Europe at least, some form of safety net for when things go wrong. The destitution of the workhouse days is gone, but deprivation—the lack of basic necessities—remains a key threat to health in the twenty-first century. We need to pay close attention to the impact of deprivation because for the last 13 years the rate at which our life expectancy increases has slowed—so much so that for the first time in a while, life expectancy has dropped. Some of this can be attributed to mortality during the COVID-19 pandemic, but as will be shown in this chapter, that same mortality has a considerable impact on the health inequalities in our society. On average, women are living 23 weeks less than they did pre-2020 (dropping from 83 years to 82.6 years) and men are living 38 weeks less (from 79.3 to 78.6 years) (Office for National Statistics, 2024). After decades of life improving from generation to generation, it is no longer the case that people will lead a healthier and longer life than the generation before them.

In this chapter, we will examine why this is the case. While medical knowledge and ability are going from strength to strength, this is no longer reflected in the health of the people receiving this medicine. This is due to the social and structural determinants of health: the socio-economic, cultural, political and environmental conditions that influence and shape the health of an individual and population.

The idea of the social (meaning the world around us) and structural (meaning the policies of that world) determinants of health is often represented by Figure 2.1 (Dahlgren and Whitehead, 1991). Nicknamed the 'Rainbow' model, it is a useful visual way to think about the main influences on health. Each 'colour' of the rainbow is a layer of influence that shapes individual health, from the overarching government policies by which we live all the way down to age and genetics. Note that even support

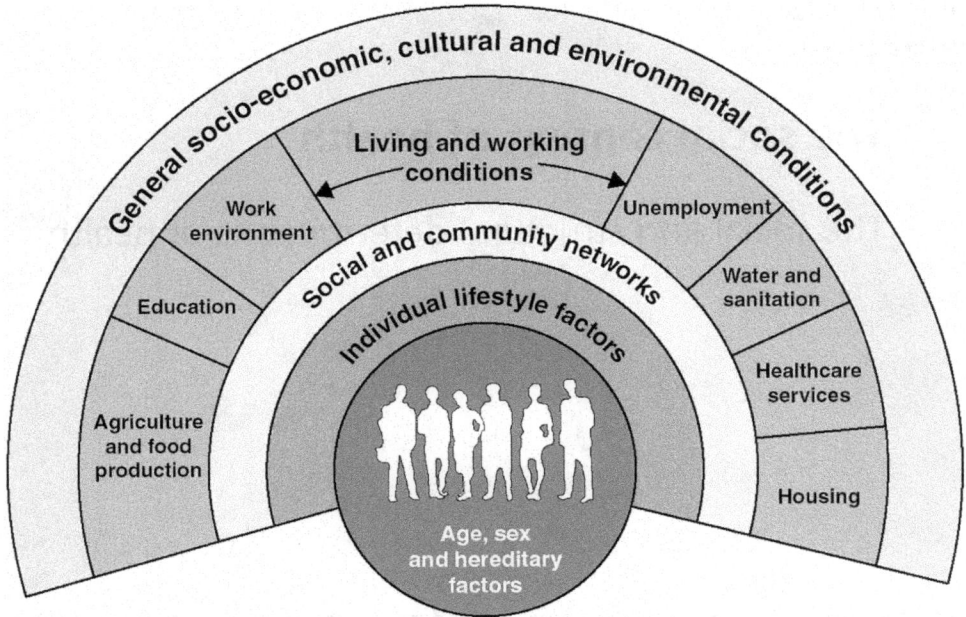

Figure 2.1 The Main Determinants of Health (Dahlgren and Whitehead, 1991).

structures are a key influence on health—indicating just how crucial the world around us really is in shaping health.

What is interesting about the determinants of health is the extent to which so much of what shapes health is external to us. For most people, there is no one big medical, genetic or scientific change that causes good or ill health. Instead, ill health is a death by a thousand everyday cuts. The determinants of health are simple things, such as where we live, work and go to school. They also include inescapable aspects of ourselves, namely our ethnicity, gender and age. While seemingly nothing to do with health, these aspects of ourselves hold different currencies in society, meaning that certain attributes, for example ethnicity or take-home pay, make us more likely to be in good or ill health. I don't want to leave you hanging, so know now that being rich and white is the best guarantee of good health in most of the world and very much so in Britain.

The differences in health that these determinants create are known as health inequalities. Health inequalities are 'the unfair and avoidable differences in health across the population, and between different groups within society' (NHS England, n.d.a). I have deliberately chosen the NHS' own definition here as it is the healthcare institution in which so many of you will be working, so it is important you understand it from that perspective. More importantly, these inequalities actually shorten people's lives and determine how healthy those lives are and even what care people can access to help support their health.

Let us take a moment to examine what is happening here and thus give some salience to why it is so important to care about the social and structural determinants of health if you work in the health profession. It is not just an interesting phenomenon; it has very real consequences. The difference in life expectancy between the least and most deprived areas in England for men, between 2020 and 2022, was ten years (Raleigh, 2024). This means that if people live in a richer area, which normally means they have the money to afford to live in that area, they are likely to live a full decade longer than someone who lives in a poorer area—which, again, normally means they have less money overall. For women, who tend to live longer than men anyway, the difference is seven years (Raleigh, 2024). These types of divides exist all over Britain and can be further detailed by healthy life expectancy, which means how long people will live in good health, not just how long they will live full stop. There is a persistent north-south divide in England with regard to living a healthy life: the healthy lifespan of those in the North East is seven (men) and six (women) years shorter than those in the South East (Raleigh, 2024). This means that these populations are spending more time in poor health and living for less time, than the equivalent populations in the South East. Just think about that the next time you contemplate a move to say, Gateshead versus Hart; you could literally be changing the length of your life. Health inequalities kill.

Inverse care law
You would think that if a particular area suffers more ill health, then there would be more healthcare facilities to help care for that population's more complex health needs. Unfortunately, you would be wrong. A perverse aspect of health inequalities is that the populations with the highest need for healthcare access tend to have the most difficulty finding that access. This is known as the inverse care law (Tudor Hart, 1971). It has three foci: the healthcare needs of the population, the access to that healthcare and the quality of the healthcare that is available (Fisher et al., 2022).

The inverse care law is not just a sad theory or scathing indictment of healthcare policy. It is the reality within which many of you will practise healthcare itself (Cookson et al., 2021; Benoit et al., 2023). This is particularly important in terms of primary and urgent care, as the areas with the most inequalities and deprivation are the areas that rely much more heavily on general practitioners (GPs) and emergency department walk-ins for healthcare. You are likely and justifiably asking yourself: how has this situation developed? Let's look at the case for general practice.

In areas affected by the inverse care law, meaning poorer areas, general practitioners have more work, larger lists and less hospital support and inherit more clinically ineffective traditions of consultation, than in the healthiest areas[1] (Fisher et al., 2022). GP practices in deprived areas also tend to have less funding and fewer doctors for their needs—and this is before we discuss how GP numbers have steadily declined since 2015, meaning that care loads are higher due to fewer doctors, regardless of where the practice is located (Fisher et al., 2022). Here, structural determinants of health are in part to blame. Despite a decades-long trend concretely showing that the inverse care law exists and has a detrimental impact on health, there have been very few policies from the government to tackle the issue. There are no requirements for vacancies to be filled or surgeries to be opened in the deprived areas that most need them. For example, if the 6,000 GPs promised by the previous Conservative government were to materialise, there is no policy in place to stop all of them going to work in wealthier areas, thus actually widening the inequalities in health that the policy was supposed to reduce (Fisher, 2021; Carey et al., 2015). Previous Labour governments made very small inroads between the 1990s and 2000s; however, with the programme of austerity set out by the Conservative government of 2010, many of these in-roads were lost, as austerity has been proven to widen inequalities (Institute of Health Equity, 2024).

Why do we have health inequalities?

To date, no government has covered themselves in glory with regards to improving health inequalities; instead there seems to be a sense of continually trying to understand where they come from and then doing absolutely nothing to tackle them. It may be that this is due to the renewed popularity in our culture of viewing health as a personal responsibility, a key characteristic of Britain's austerity years (2010–2024). Alternatively, COVID-19 and the cost-of-living crisis may have drawn these inequalities into such stark relief that governments can no longer justify ignoring them completely. The real reason is unclear; likely, as with most things relating to the social and structural determinants of health, it is a bit of both.

What is odd—and perhaps a sort of voyeurism care law if you will indulge me—is that for well over 50 years, Britain has been aware of health inequalities; for at least 40 of those years it has been trying to ascertain what causes them. Humour me in a brief meander through the many ways that health inequalities are thought to develop and why some of these are utter nonsense.

By 1977, six years after GP Julian Tudor Hart coined the term *inverse care law*, the Labour government had commissioned Sir Douglas Black to chair a 'working group on inequalities in health' (The Health Foundation, n.d.). The goal was to investigate why different areas and populations had different health outcomes and come up with some reasons why this had happened. In yet another example of society influencing health, by the time the group was ready to publish in 1980, the Labour party was out and Thatcher was in, meaning that the recommendations were never acted on as they were considered too expensive by her government (The Health Foundation, n.d.). The working group published their findings in August 1980 under the title *Inequalities in health: report of a research working group*, though it has been known as the 'Black Report' for most of its existence. It confirmed that health inequalities did exist and posited four possible explanations for health inequalities. (As a point of historical interest, the report cost £8 to access. In today's money that is about £35, meaning someone would have to work for about four hours at the current 18–20 year old minimum wage of £8.60 an hour just to be able to read the thing (Socialist Health Association, 2012). Even today there continues to be a disconnect in politics between reports about people and the people themselves, but I digress.)

The four possible reasons for health inequalities suggested by the Black Report were:

1. Artefact explanation
2. Natural and social selection
3. Cultural/behavioural explanation
4. Materialist or structural explanation (considered to be the most likely explanation for health inequalities)

Let us briefly consider each one.

The artefact explanation argued that health inequalities were perhaps not real. Instead, health inequalities arose due to the way statistics were collected for social status, for example the way information was collected on occupational class. This meant that health inequalities were effectively a measurement error. This is largely a discredited explanation of health inequalities. In fact, it is likely that measurement error at the time actually concealed the true extent of health inequalities, thus causing policy-makers to underestimate their impact on the health of the population (McCartney at al., 2013). Perhaps the best lasting legacy of this debunked theory is the effort to capture social status better in future statistical measuring of the population.

The natural and social selection theory has also been discarded as a possible cause of health inequalities. Here, the argument is that being sick moves people down in social status. It is not that people low on the social rungs have worse health, but that becoming ill lowers this status. Sick individuals move down the social hierarchy; healthy individuals move up. Perhaps this is true to a very small extent. It is hard to deny that in British culture, chronically ill and disabled people are more likely to be disadvantaged; however, later studies have suggested that, at most, social selection makes only a minor contribution to the huge socio-economic differentials in health and mortality. The theory fails to account for the many people born into lower social status who never slide down the social pole, but are still more likely to have poor health over their lifetimes (Blane et al., 1993).

The cultural/behavioural explanation once again relates to our old friend, personal responsibility in health. This theory argues that ill health is due to people's choices, which are shaped by their knowledge and goals. The uncharitable way of viewing this, and I am going to be uncharitable, is that the stupider someone is, the less they know about good health, and so they will make bad choices for themself out of ignorance that result in both ill health and having less money (Socialist Health Association, n.d.). Let's just leave a space around that while we all scream our frustration into the void at the ignorance of that theory.

A more refined and professional take on the cultural/behavioural explanation is that people from disadvantaged backgrounds tend to engage in more health-damaging behaviours, while people from advantaged backgrounds tend to engage in more health-promoting behaviours. This might be a useful explanation to justify health education campaigns, but it has serious limitations. As we have already seen, behaviours are not individual choices made in a vacuum; instead, they are the outcomes of social processes and contexts. The choices available to people in different socio-economic groups are almost always vastly different and grossly unequal, meaning that people in lower socio-economic groups are often left in a 'best house on a bad block' situation when making choices. It hardly seems fair to say this is somehow their fault when they can only choose from the choices genuinely available to them.

A campaign by Cancer Research UK from a few years ago is a great example of why the cultural/behavioural explanation gets it so wrong. In 2018, Cancer Research UK caused considerable controversy by taking out tube station adverts and billboards with the tagline: 'OB_S__Y: Guess what is the biggest preventable cause of cancer after smoking' (Bodkin and Horton, 2018).

It caused quite a stir, and this was in large part due to the total black and white approach (literally and figuratively) it took to the role that obesity plays in cancer prevention. Obesity might cause cancer, but what causes obesity? Let me tell you. One of the biggest preventable causes of obesity is inequality and poverty (Adams, 2020). In England, adults in the most deprived neighbourhoods are almost twice as likely to be obese as those in the least deprived neighbourhoods (NHS England, 2019). Healthy food is expensive, gym memberships are expensive, areas of deprivation (in which people on lower incomes often find themselves living) are often more urban with less outdoor space for exercising and that space may not be safe (Adams, 2020). Lower income groups often take shift work, working odd hours and permanent nights (among other factors). To frame obesity as a willing choice that people make that leads to cancer lays the blame for illness on those least able to make the choices that would avoid obesity. To paraphrase Adams, who has done a fair bit of research on this, it is not because poor people are lazy gluttons with no self-restraint that they are also more likely to be fat (Adams, 2020).[2]

Twitter users were not impressed by the campaign either. It remains unconfirmed, though never denied, that the British Psychological Society ran a response campaign on Twitter with the tagline: 'P_V_RTY: Guess what is a major preventable cause of early death?' (Feminist Rewrites, 2018).

Regardless of who was really behind this post, I would argue it is a better advertising campaign as it considers both health and social influences. With our obesity example, while it is absolutely correct that medicine can pinpoint scientific reasons why obesity increases a person's chance of developing cancer, understanding why someone is obese to begin with is as important as pointing out this health risk. Obesity is not a wilful choice; as reams of social science research over recent decades has shown, obesity is very often the by-product of a person's socio-economic context and the health inequalities they have to live with as a result of that context (Adams, 2020). Not considering a person's lack of access to the necessary tools to lose weight due to their social context is the equivalent of prescribing a drug to a patient that isn't available in the United Kingdom: useless and ineffective medical practice. This is why health inequalities and socio-economic context matter so much in health, not only when we create health policy but also at the sharp end, when a doctor has a patient sitting in front of them. They have to consider not just which treatment is best, but which of the treatment options the patient can best access.

So, what causes health inequalities? You are dying to know and I've strung you along for several theories now. Lest you think the Black Report was just killing time on the government's dime, they did develop the most plausible and longest-lasting explanation for health inequalities: what they called the Material or Structural Explanation. I prefer the Structural Explanation and it is my book, so that is what we are going to call it.

The structural explanation for health inequalities

The Structural Explanation argues that differences in socio-economic circumstances create differences in health outcomes (Socialist Health Association, n.d.; McCartney et al., 2013). These differences in socio-economic circumstances relate to the access that individuals and communities have to resources such as overall wealth, power, household income and environment. The more resources someone has, the more power they have over the choices available to them, such as where they live, what they do for work, what they eat and the activities in which they take part. This leads to an overall healthier life. On top of this, the positive or negative impact of a person's access to these resources actually accumulates throughout their life. This means that if they have fewer resources available to them, they will likely rack up more ill health over their lifetime—this might include worsening conditions, more chronic disease, a lower life expectancy or all three—than if they had more resources available to them (Marmot et al., 2010).

The Structural Explanation for health inequalities has been proven over and over again by the available data. The explanation is able to explain not just why we have ill health, but why we have good health. When structural inequalities are reduced in a community (often by chance), the health of the whole community improves as a result (Krieger et al., 2008; Thomas et al., 2010; Costello et al., 2003). The reverse is true too. Where there are more structural inequalities, health becomes worse. For example, the Marmot Report of 2010, *Fair Society, Healthy Lives* (Marmot et al., 2010), showed that when looking at area deprivation, a good indicator of structural inequalities and availability of resources, it could be seen that 70% of people living in the least deprived areas had no health conditions at all. In contrast, among those living in the most deprived areas, 75% had one health condition, 50% at least two and 25% had three or more health conditions (Marmot et al., 2010, figure 10).

Before you go down the personal responsibility route that so many people like to take when condemning the health and health behaviours of those living in deprivation, remember that we have already debunked this myth when we dismissed the cultural explanation for health inequalities. If you need further convincing that it does not just boil down to poorer people making poorer decisions about their health, you may be interested to know that if someone has better access to material resources (i.e. more money), they are more likely to be in good health than someone with fewer resources (i.e. less money) REGARDLESS of the health behaviours they engage in (World Health Organisation, 2008). In fact, the relationship between health and wealth is so strong that it even persists where genetic factors, such as mutations that cause disease, are the cause of ill health, showing just how strong social and structural determinants are in shaping health (Barr et al., 2011).

Since the Black Report, there have been other, equally damning, reports showing that health inequalities have only continued to grow in Britain. Both of the Marmot Reports (2010 and 2020) showed this to be a clear trend (Marmot et al., 2010, 2020). There are two additional theories since the Black Report that have added more detail to the Structural Explanation for health inequalities; I would like to touch on these before moving on to look at real world examples of health inequality.

The psychosocial explanation is one theory. Here, the argument is that inequalities in health are not necessarily due to the actual differences in people's income (i.e. socio-economic status), but the direct and indirect stress we feel because of where we find ourselves in the socio-economic hierarchy (Marmot and Wilkinson, 2001). The psychosocial theory tries to capture the impact of stressors and stress on health. In particular, it focuses on the way social factors can influence our state of mind and health. The psychosocial explanation is a double whammy for health inequalities: it is not just a person's access (or lack thereof) to resources that influences their health, but the psychosocial variables related to that access, such as anxiety, insecurity, control and depression. Together, all of these make the difference between good and ill health (Marmot and Wilkinson, 2001). Over the years, this theory has been debated as to the extent to which it can truly account for all health inequalities, but it likely has some validity. Stressors in life are known to impact our biology, as we saw earlier in our discussion of epigenetics. It is also hard to deny that things like trauma can have a profound and lasting influence on people's lives, which translates into lifelong consequences for their physical and mental health (Bell, 2017). As such, the psychosocial explanation is likely part of the explanation for at least some individuals and communities.

Another theory that has been put forth since the Black Report is that of Income Distribution. Developed by Wilkinson, who worked with Marmot on the psychosocial theory (there is some overlap between the two), the Income Distribution theory suggests that countries with more unequal distribution of wealth will also have greater health inequalities (Wilkinson, 1990). Wilkinson posited that this is because life expectancy tends to be highest in countries where income is more equally distributed (Wilkinson, 1990), which is a damning indictment of capitalism's effect on world health. Both of these theories are variations on a theme: trying to understand why health inequalities should exist at all in countries where, for the most part, the most basic of needs (water, sanitation, healthcare) are met. It is very clear, regardless of the theory, that the more unequal other aspects are in an area, the more likely health inequalities will exist there.

Health inequalities in the real world: how the social and structural determinants of health caused the opioid crisis in the United States

There is no arguing that there are health inequalities in our societies. We have some idea as to why they exist, but how influential are they really? They make for interesting statistics and shocking figures, but can they really change health that much? Yes—and the answer lies in better understanding the structural determinants of health. A big part of what makes up society is its governance: the laws, policies and practices it has around most things, including health. These are the structural determinants of health we discussed at the beginning of the chapter, and they are one of the key reasons we have health inequalities in the first place. To understand this better, we will cross the pond to the United States and look at what I believe to be one of the most tragic health inequalities-related emergencies caused by structural determinants of health in the twenty-first century: the opioid crisis.

For several years there has been a recognised relationship between opioid (mis)use, mortality and social determinants of health (Albright et al., 2021). In certain deprived areas, such as the Appalachian Region of the United States, there is a higher rate of opioid prescription and (mis)use (Levy et al., 2015). It has been recognised that communities in this area have structural inequalities that negatively impact their health, such as lack of access to healthcare due to financial constraints. This likely stems from the area having high levels of unemployment/poorly paid employment (Albright et al., 2021), which has in turn been linked to the increased use of opioids.[3] Several studies have also linked key inequalities, such as unstable housing, lack of secondary education and employment status to opioid use (Albright et al., 2021; Nicholson, 2020).

What does this tell us? First, that people with less education, a bad housing situation and a low-paid and/or inconsistent job are more likely to be using opioids. When we unpack these three indicators, this is not a surprise. Education levels are linked to employment. Across the world, the higher a person's education, the more likely they are to be employed (OECD, 2020). The more likely they are to be employed, the more likely they are to have stable housing, and interestingly, the other way around too (Moisi, 2020). A causal relationship is forming here, and you would be forgiven for thinking that if people just stayed in education, there would be no opioid crisis.

But, as with everything in this book, it is not that simple.

When we dive deeper into policies in the United States, we learn more about exactly how the opioid crisis arose; it has little to do with the addicts.

A few basics first.

Prescription opioids are used to treat pain—usually acute pain from cancer. The kind of pain that floors a person and keeps them there for a while. You might be interested, or at the very least shocked, to hear that the United States has no federal laws requiring employers to provide sick leave—paid or unpaid (US Department of Labor, n.d.). Only 15 out of the 50 states have laws protecting and providing sick leave (Weston Williamson, 2024). Private and civil employers can choose to provide some sort of sick leave, but they are not legally compelled to do so and it can be unpaid if they want it to be. This means that, in some jobs, people can be fired for taking a day (or several in the case of cancer) off work for illness. This is a pretty extreme example, but still possible, especially in states that allow 'at-will employment', which allows an employee to be fired (or quit) for any reason at any time (Cornell Law School, n.d.)—so long as they are not fired for an unlawful reason, which does not always include illness. Different employers, cities and states have different rules around this, but the standard offering for sick leave in the United States is an average of seven days after one year in the job (US Department of Labor, 2019). Don't worry—this rises to a whopping EIGHT days after 20 years of service (US Department of Labor, 2019). An individual's ability to take time off work if ill or injured is thus directly dependent on their employment contract and where they live.

Of course, the lowest earners in the United States, such as those in the Appalachian Region, have the least access to paid sick leave (US Department of Labor, 2023). Only half of food service, accommodation, leisure and hospitality employees have access to such leave (Weston Williamson, 2024). Seasonal workers are also often left without any sick pay or leave entitlement at all, as many employers require at least 90 days continual employment before they will extend benefits to their employees (Leiwant et al., 2019). In Appalachia, to return to our case study, the most common work (now that mining is in decline in the region) is in food, accommodation and leisure (Appalachian Regional Commission, 2011)—the jobs with only a 50% chance of paid sick leave. It also lags behind the rest of the United States in employment more generally (US Department of Labor, 2022), which is no surprise; as recently as 13 years ago, only 12% of adults had a college education in Central Appalachia (Appalachian Regional Commission, 2011) compared to 27.5% in the rest of the country. It is also much harder to access affordable healthcare and treatment in the region, resulting in higher rates of common diseases such as cancer, heart disease and diabetes (Appalachian Regional Commission, 2011).

To recap the relevant details of the Appalachian Region's opioid crisis: there is a policy landscape that does not protect an individual when they are most vulnerable, in a population likely to be in low-paying employment where voluntary benefits are not offered to staff and living in a deprived environment characterised by ill health and a lack of post-secondary education. All of this is happening in a country that does not support universal healthcare for its population and has a very complex and often useless set of health and social care laws.

A perfect storm in terms of social and structural determinants of health. But it doesn't end there. Social and cultural norms inform and are informed by policy.

Perhaps due to the difficulty of taking time off work for ill health, American doctors like to prescribe drugs. They do it all the time. The American culture is characterised by an expectation from both doctors and patients that a drug will be prescribed as part of the interaction between them (Garber, 2019). Additionally, basic healthcare benefits will often pay for pills but not for more complex treatment such as physiotherapy or surgery (Amos, 2017). So we now add a willingness and expectation to prescribe pills and the need to use pills as an alternative to better clinical care to the already swirling determinant storm that requires sick people to work when they should be trying to get better. All of this together means that the Appalachian community need and want a quick and a cheap way to deal with the pain, so they can return to whatever job they currently have, while they still have it. The situation becomes even more complex. We cannot simply pin the prescription opioid crisis on poor people trying to get back into work. Larger structural forces are at play, and they have devastating health consequences.

Against this backdrop of a prescription drug culture and a lack of protected sick leave, research has found that about half of all doctors who prescribe opioids in the United States receive some sort of money from pharma companies in return. This is completely legal (Kessler et al., 2018). Policy allows this to happen within a set of rules that the pharma companies know inside and out. Often this is in the form of paid speeches to promote the drug—nothing as obvious as a kick-back, but, as was uncovered seven years ago, the more a doctor prescribes an opioid, the more likely they are to be making money from it in other ways (Kessler et al., 2018). Additionally, the Food and Drug Administration (FDA), the regulatory body for medicine in the United States, has limited powers in certain areas such as drug promotion and marketing (US Food and Drug Administration, 2015). In fact, they have no power to limit the amount of money spent on marketing a drug. Drug companies can pay current prescribers to hold talks, train other professionals and provide consulting services on the particular drugs that these companies want doctors to prescribe. Those within a profession tend to trust each other, and so they see no reason to doubt a fellow healthcare professional who tells them about a great new drug they have found for their patients. The conflict of interest is clear, but from a policy point of view, this is considered completely acceptable. As shocking as it may seem, commercial interests are frequently put ahead of health; this was (and still is, really) the case for opioid use in the United States. Let me follow up with another example, as this will help to illustrate a key structural determinant of health while also providing the final piece of the puzzle that shows how the opioid crisis is actually a social, cultural and political crisis.

Oxycontin, Purdue and the curious case of the commercial determinants of health

One determinant of health that is not always discussed is the commercial determinant of health. Commercial determinants of health are activities in the private sector, that is areas and industries that make money, that directly and indirectly influence health in positive and negative ways (World Health Organisation, 2023). The influence and impact of commercial determinants of health are very wide-ranging; they can be anything from a packaging choice that impacts the lived environment to lobbying for a change that positively impacts an industry but not necessarily the health of those engaging in that industry. I consider it a subset of the structural determinants of health because commercial interests, like social and cultural behaviours and beliefs, do not exist in a vacuum. Instead, most commercial determinants of health are completely legal within the policy framework of the country where they operate. In short, even if they are harming health, they are allowed to engage in such activity if it abides by the laws of the country. As policy and law are aspects of the structural determinants of health, this arguably makes commercial determinants of health an aspect within structural determinants. Incidentally, structural determinants are both the cause and solution to the negative impact of commercial determinants of health, as only a change in policy can stop a practice that is affecting our health (Gilmore et al., 2023).

In 1996, Purdue Pharma introduced its prescription opioid drug, OxyContin, to the market. OxyContin is an excellent example of the commercial determinants of health and a cautionary tale of why the structural and social determinants of health need to be ever-present in the mind of the modern healthcare professional. Prescription opioids had been around for some time; however, due to various issues with side effects and the risk of addiction, they were only used to treat people with acute pain such as cancer patients and those at the end of life (NHS England, n.d.b). Opioid use for cancer pain control is a relatively small market, as not everyone needs opioids and those who do tend to use them for short periods of time—what we call acute pain relief (Van Zee, 2009). But chronic pain is just that: long-term. Forever. It is a huge market where massive sums of money can be made, and Purdue wanted in on that market. Taking advantage of the more relaxed policies around opioid use for pain that had been introduced in the 1990s (Van Zee, 2009), Purdue aggressively marketed their drug, OxyContin, for the long-term control of chronic pain, falsely claiming that OxyContin was non-addictive (Van Zee, 2009). In doing so, they started a trend for prescription opioid use in chronic pain. By 1999, just three years later, the non-cancer-related pain market represented 86% of the opioid market (*Oxycontin Marketing Plan*, 2001; Van Zee, 2009).

To this day, there exists almost no credible evidence that prescription opioids are a better choice for chronic pain relief (Royal College of Anaesthetists, n.d.). The decision to pursue this drug in this way was a commercial one—it was made to make Purdue Pharma as much money as they could in an under-utilised market. Despite the clear and solid evidence provided to the FDA that OxyContin was no more effective than the existing opioids of the time for acute pain, the lack of governance around marketing (i.e. a structural determinant of health) allowed Purdue to pour as much money as they wanted into the promotion of the drug, and they did. By 2002, the prescription rate of OxyContin had increased tenfold (Government Accountability Office, 2003). These policies allowed Purdue to misrepresent the risk of addiction to OxyContin by claiming the addiction rate for its drug was 'less than one per cent', when those numbers actually came from acute pain studies where use was neither long-term nor in chronic pain sufferers (Van Zee, 2009; Meier, 2003). In reality, rates of addiction in chronic pain sufferers who used opioids were sometimes as high as 50% 11 years after OxyContin's release (Højsted and Sjøgren, 2007). More recently, estimates are still high, with 29% of users becoming addicted (Vowles et al., 2015). In contrast, addiction rates in cancer patients have remained consistently lower, even at the height of the opioid crisis (Højsted and Sjøgren, 2007).

It was not just government policies around advertising and the advertising itself that made the drug such a juggernaut. Key to OxyContin's popularity was that it is a relatively inexpensive drug; it was marketed as effective for common chronic pain injuries such as back pain, and an OxyContin prescription was normally covered even by basic healthcare (National Drug Intelligence Center, 2001). This appealed to people in more deprived areas (Congressional Budget Office, 2022) who were looking to medicate themselves cheaply against conditions that either they could not afford to treat further or their health insurance would not cover (Amos, 2017). In other words, because those in lower socio-economic groups had less access to the resources they needed to access healthcare (the structural explanation for health inequalities), they were obligated to choose a less optimal, but more easily accessible, treatment to meet their health needs (health inequalities as a result of the negative impact of the structural and social determinants of health) (Moody et al., 2017).

This is how we end up with pockets of extreme misuse like the Appalachian Region. It was the perfect environment within which to market and prescribe the drug. It is likely that doctors may have even felt they were doing their patients a great service by prescribing what they thought was a non-addictive, long-term pain relief drug that their patients could afford, as it allowed them to carry on with their everyday lives (Appalachian Regional Commission, 2019) in a region prone to injury in jobs and insecure jobs (Moody et al., 2017). Instead, it started a cascade of addiction that plagues the region even today (Appalachian Regional Commission, 2019). Despite a recognised above-national-average rate of addiction and death, access to healthcare in the region, especially public health measures to support and control addiction, remains limited (Appalachian Regional Commission, 2019). Additionally, the personal responsibility approach to medicine adopted in the United States creates a policy environment that is unlikely to be supportive of those in need. Indeed, policy has done little to help this area, which is already deprived, and as a result, life expectancy in Appalachia has remained consistently lower than the nation in general for well over two decades (Woodard, 2023). Incidentally, those two decades correspond with the rise of the opioid crisis.

I have told you this story because it shows you how a collection of 'non-clinical' phenomena—a bunch of policies, practices and beliefs related to health—can work together, effectively destroying the good health of an entire community. This is why it is so important to keep the structural explanation for health inequalities in your mind when you see patients. The route by which they ended up in need of your care in the first place may be very complex, and the solution may have very little to do with clinical care—though clinical care will likely help. Your patients are the sum of their parts, with their parts being that triad from chapter one: their biological selves, their psychological selves and their social selves. Each must be addressed because each is acted on by the world around them and so each plays a part in the overall health of a person or community.

Health inequities

So far, we have looked at how health inequalities, caused by the social, structural and commercial determinants of health, create unfair and avoidable differences in health across a population. However, there are also systemic differences that act on different groups within that population and create further disparities in health. Systemic differences in health are those differences caused by the system: meaning the social, cultural, legal, political and economic world in which we live. The impact of racism on health is a good example of health inequity and the systemic determinants of health, which is why we will examine the concept through the lens of racism in Britain.

First, here are a few important and basic facts about racism more generally and its impact on the United Kingdom. Racism limits where people can live, work, go to school and how and to what extent they access healthcare (Ray, 2023; Paton et al., 2020; Benoit et al., 2023). This creates poor health outcomes for people from ethnic backgrounds;[4] these outcomes are unjust and avoidable—meaning they would not exist if these groups were treated the same as white British people. This is health inequity— systemic differences in access to healthcare that causes unfair and avoidable poor health outcomes for certain communities or groups of people.

Take the relationship between racism and housing. We already know that housing is important for good health, as we saw this in our discussion of the opioid crisis. Stable housing also supports job stability. Good health prevents disease and improves overall quality of life (World Health Organisation, 2018). In fact, housing is probably one of the most researched social determinants of health. Policy may ignore this relationship, but it is an uncontroversial and accepted relationship that good housing means good health (Taylor, 2018).

However, access to good housing is limited by current and historic racism in the United Kingdom. More than half of Black tenants (56%) are denied the right to a safe home, and almost as many (49%) Asian tenants are in the same boat (Shelter, n.d.). Black households are 11 times more likely to be living in temporary housing than white households, and 23% of people seeking help for homelessness are from an ethnic background (Shelter, n.d.). The fact that this number is disproportionately high, given that only 14% of ALL households identify as being from an ethnic background, tells us that the disparity is likely due to discrimination.

Why is this the case at all, given that the United Kingdom is made up of various ethnicities with diverse and culturally unique communities all over the country? Well, Britain's inglorious colonial history has a lot to answer for here (King, 2021). I am not going to entertain a discussion of whether British colonialism was a positive or negative political and historical force. The British bulldozed their way into other countries and declared them their own, treating the local populations appallingly—all while trying to argue it was more civilised to sweat in brogues and tweed while sipping tea than to bother understanding the practices and cultures of colonised countries who had done just fine for centuries before the British arrived. The legacy of colonialism in health, as in most things, is one of slavery, racism, betrayal and, for our purposes, health inequity.

In Britain, racism lives on as part of that colonial legacy even today. It has impacted every part of life for people of colour. Even when people from former and current colonies arrived to help in post-WWII Britain, they were met with prejudice and excluded from proper housing and secure jobs (King, 2021). This has had a generations-long impact on Black and Asian communities in Britain in particular. As a result, people of colour are today more likely to live in densely populated urban areas and in overcrowded accommodations (Paton et al., 2020). Around 50% of Pakistani, Bangladeshi, Black African and Black Caribbean communities live in the two most deprived deciles of the country (Paton et al., 2020). This means that these communities are likely to be in worse housing and thus in worse health for no other reason than their skin colour.

If you are thinking that this is deeply messed up, you are right. Just wait until you hear about how racism affected this population's health during a world crisis. Let's look at my own work on health inequity through the lens of housing, racism, health and the COVID-19 pandemic.

COVID-19 and racism: a case study in health inequity

Very early on in the COVID-19 pandemic, it became clear from the data that healthcare staff from ethnic backgrounds were more likely to die of COVID than white British staff (Paton et al., 2020). It then became clear that patients from ethnic backgrounds were experiencing worse outcomes and dying in higher numbers than white patients (Paton et al., 2020). COVID was clearly dangerous and deadly for people who were not white. There are a number of reasons why this is the case, but let's stay focused on housing for now.

We already know that people from ethnic backgrounds are more likely to live in urban environments that are overcrowded and located in more deprived areas. Public health measures at the time of the COVID-19 pandemic were focused on staying home and controlling the spread (Paton, 2022). However, that is tricky to do when living in an overcrowded, multigenerational home where ventilation and isolation are impossible. Additionally, these deprived urban environments, where almost half of people of colour in the United Kingdom live, are known to have poor air quality, which has been associated with poorer outcomes from COVID-19 (Paton et al., 2020). The result of the racist beliefs and policies from Britain's history is that people of colour were (and still are) living in areas that were more likely to make them sick and less able to follow public health advice to try and avoid infection compared to the equivalent white population (Paton et al., 2020). Modern day public health policies, which were supposed to protect the population as a whole, failed to account for the fact that these communities often could not take these precautions to the extent necessary for meaningful mitigation of the virus. This is a direct example of the way health inequities cause disparities in health that otherwise would not exist. This is how deeply unfair our society is and how that unfairness is literally killing certain members of society—and we have only looked at housing.

I suspect you understand my point and agree with me, but I'll go on because it is my book and I have an important point to make here. We will look at the role occupation played in COVID-19 next. There is a similar story to tell; people of colour were at greater risk and were dying in bigger numbers than white people doing the same jobs. Over 40% of doctors, dentists and consultants and almost 30% of nurses, midwives and health visitors are from ethnic backgrounds (NHS England, 2023). In fact, about a quarter of all NHS staff comes from an ethnic background (NHS England, 2023). This is important because, as early as April 2020—only one month after the pandemic was even declared—an estimated 64% of COVID-19 related deaths were healthcare workers from ethnic backgrounds (Paton et al., 2020). Broken down by major profession, 71% of nurses, 56% of support staff and 94% of doctors/dentists who died from COVID-19 in this first month came from ethnic backgrounds. In addition, staff from ethnic backgrounds are over-represented in the transport and distribution and retail sectors (Paton et al., 2020). Employees from these sectors continued to work and interact face-to-face with the public throughout the pandemic. Analysis of COVID-19-related deaths among ethnic populations within these sectors remains underdeveloped, but is likely to match the unequal impact seen in the healthcare sector (Paton et al., 2020).

Not only are people from ethnic backgrounds more exposed to the risk of infection, but they also tend to work more precarious jobs and are less likely to work from home (Paton et al., 2020). Employment dictates how much money we have to spend on important things such as housing, food and warmth—all of which contribute to good or ill health. For a population already at risk, losing a job dramatically increases the likelihood of ending up in ill health. In the workplace, people from ethnic backgrounds were at greater risk than their white counterparts; this is extremely problematic. It sends a social, cultural and political message that ethnic communities do not matter as much as white communities: that their deaths are more acceptable when they are not. This is especially galling because, without staff from ethnic backgrounds, the health and social care systems in the United Kingdom would likely fall apart, such is their importance to the successful running of both.

Despite the important role that staff from ethnic backgrounds play in the NHS, our clinical policies and practices also contribute to health inequities for this group. We know from previous pandemics that when decision tools emphasise certain clinical markers, specifically long-term survival and co-morbidity, to determine priority of care, the resulting prioritisation decisions around clinical care disproportionately disadvantage people from ethnic backgrounds (Daugherty Biddeson et al., 2019). This is because people of colour are more likely to have the health conditions that these decision tools deem to be inappropriate for critical care (Paton et al., 2020). This is most often due to health inequities and inequalities caused by the social and structural determinants of health (Ray, 2023)—that is factors completely outside of their control.

One example of this is the focus on cardiovascular co-morbidities in the 'Information to support decision making' document released by NICE during the first COVID-19 wave (NICE, 2020). The document explicitly singled out angina as a co-morbidity (meaning that someone has more than one disease at the same time) that should be used to determine whether a patient was a candidate for escalation of care (NICE, 2020). It may have made sense on the surface, but for people of South Asian background, who are at a higher risk of cardiovascular problems such as angina, this was terrifying grounds on which they could be denied treatment during the pandemic (British Heart Foundation, n.d.). The focus on cardiovascular co-morbidities is just one of dozens of examples of people of colour not receiving the same care as white British patients. Health emergencies where people of colour are more likely to die happen time and time again (Daugherty Biddeson et al., 2019). We KNOW that this type of focus in a health emergency creates these inequities and leads to unjust deaths, and yet policy and practice forge on ahead, pretending their hands are tied. This is yet another example of health inequity, where access to healthcare itself is unequal but the inequality is also avoidable. By failing to account for the relationship between ethnicity and health, the existing guidance, among so many other policies and practices, actually widens health inequalities and inequities overall (Paton, 2022). Another pandemic is a forgone conclusion, but there is now an opportunity to develop policies that are less destructive to communities of people of colour in Britain before that happens.

Gender and health: the final nail in the coffin of health equality and health equity

There is a recognised relationship between gender and health. You may have heard, and even used, the old adage 'Men die quicker, but women get sicker'. It is true that on average, women live longer than men and that they tend to live that longer life with more non-fatal illnesses (Patwardhan et al., 2024). Women's lives are marked by mental illness and conditions that cause pain, whereas men are much more likely to contract fatal illnesses such as heart problems or die suddenly from road injuries and acute illness such as COVID-19 (Patwardhan et al., 2024). These differences persist with age, meaning they stay with and often get worse as women age; as such, women live longer with higher rates of illness and disability then men (Patwardhan et al., 2024). There are some possible biological differences that help explain the gender gap in health, but they are minimal and not the focus of this book. Furthermore, closer investigation makes it obvious that many of these biological differences are very much due to the social world, not the medical (Vlassoff, 2007), and the biological differences that should matter have been steadfastly ignored by science.

I would like to end this chapter with a discussion of the gender health gap and why it is an important concept to understand in order to practise good medicine. What is interesting about this health gap is that it brings together social norms around gender, expectations within a community or culture around expected gender roles, the overall policy ethos of the country where an individual lives and the consequences of pretending to be 'gender blind' in clinical and scientific work (or simply not bothering to study women at all—we will get to that). The gender health gap is a kaleidoscope of social and structural determinants, combined with scientific bias, which creates both inequalities and inequities in health.

We have spent some time discussing policy and health equity, so we will start there. Gender health inequalities are wider in countries where there are no policies attempting to reduce gender inequity more generally (SOPHIE Project, n.d.). For example, in southern and central Europe (i.e. Portugal, Spain, France, Belgium, the Netherlands and Germany), the policy models fail to promote gender equity, as they reflect what we would call 'traditional' societal norms, where women are not the primary earners in the family (SOPHIE Project, n.d.). Women in these regions are expected to take on substantial care roles in their families, and there are few family support policies that would provide greater equity in the family and workplace (SOPHIE Project, n.d.). As a result, women in these countries report higher levels of ill health than men, both physical and mental (SOPHIE Project, n.d.). Policy can turn this around. When countries have explicit policies in place to address these differences, such as better support for family care and societal expectations of an equal distribution of labour between genders, as is the case in Scandinavian countries, women report fewer issues with their health overall and participate more equally in life and work (SOPHIE Project, n.d.).

These differences in health persist across socio-economic status, though in general, ill health is more pronounced for women who have less money, are from an ethnic background and/or are immigrants (SOPHIE Project, n.d.). This is called the intersectionality of health. Intersectionality is a framework, a way of understanding how the different aspects of someone's life come together or 'intersect' to influence their health, including the way that the systems of oppression and power under which they live limit that life (Crenshaw, 1989). It is a way to understand better how discrimination develops and what that means for the people experiencing that discrimination. As a concept, intersectionality can help identify systemic changes that can reduce the impact of discrimination or even remove it all together (Routen et al., 2023). This is all a prolonged way of saying that we could easily eliminate the gender health gap by making it a policy priority globally. Needless to say, as a general rule, that is yet to happen.

Beyond policy and messed-up societal and social media ideals about what a woman 'should be', medicine has a lot to answer for in terms of reinforcing the gender health gap by actively promoting the gender data gap (Criado Pérez, 2019). Clinical and medical research has, for the most part, focused exclusively on men (Merone et al., 2022). The reason for this exclusion is the outdated and misogynistic social and cultural norms about women that still persist. Women have been viewed as either too important, as a reproductive vessel, to risk harming in a clinical study or too busy caring for their family to have time for involvement in such things. The attitude is all very Handmaid's Tale. Men have been viewed—and this really boggles the mind here—as a 'neutral' entity on which to perform research, despite being so significantly different biologically from women that this makes absolutely no scientific sense at all (Fox, 2023; Beery and Zucker, 2011). Considering that most clinical research is so pernickety as to express a preference for the type of mouse used, lest the wrong kind interrupt the experimental process, it hardly seems a strong argument that men are somehow the neutral option when women make up half of the human population.[5] Information on medication, clinical criteria for diagnosis and treatment of major disease and illness are all designed around data that was either collected exclusively from men or not gender-disaggregated (meaning that it could have worked for women, but when mixed in with the data from men, the intervention or drug was deemed clinically ineffective (Criado Pérez, 2019) because it failed to work for both men and women). This means that it is harder to treat women effectively because the guidance for diagnosis and the recommended treatments have not been specifically tested to ensure that they are effective for women (Criado Pérez, 2019). More shockingly, to choose just one example, there are strong scientific and clinical arguments for researching women's health needs separately due to the difference in the hormone levels in women's bodies and how they change dramatically as women age (Fox, 2023; Hammes, 2024).

The result? Women are spending more time in ill health waiting for diagnosis, are more likely to have adverse drug effects when taking medication and can even have worse health outcomes due to delays from misdiagnosis and simply being downright ignored by medicine when they report illness in the first place (Bailey, 2023). The last example is called 'Yentl Syndrome', after the Barbra Streisand movie and a nineteenth century novel that most of us will never read; basically, it is when doctors only take women's symptoms seriously if they match up to known ones in men (Healy, 1991). Some days I just can't with medicine. This is before we even start with women of colour or trans women, who, it seems, do not even exist in the clinical research world outside of a select few speciality areas.

All of this shows just how critical it is as a healthcare professional for you to understand the inherent gaps in your own knowledge, how they will undoubtedly bias you in the care you give and how you yourself will unwittingly perpetuate health inequity and inequality in your own career. Even female healthcare professionals will fall foul of this because they are limited by the knowledge passed on in medicine that remains heavily reliant on information exclusively for and about men. This is known as the 'hidden curriculum' in medicine (Rajput et al., 2017) and it persists to this day. You have probably already been in a lecture this week where this has happened—as it will the next week and the one after that. This is why knowledge of the way the social world impacts all aspects of health is so vital for good healthcare. Without it, you only have half the story, and even then, as this section has shown, for only half the people under your care.

Conclusion

The fact that the world we live in has such a profound influence on our health should not be such a foreign concept in medicine as it is. We accept that the world can cause us injury, that it can infect us, even kill us, yet only in the most basic of ways. We can trip on a rock, we can pick up a virus from an unclean surface and we can die from a bear attack. Our world is not benign. The social and structural determinants of health show us just how deadly even societal beliefs can be—how the policy of a country can change the life course of a whole community. The fact that some people are healthier than others is not due to chance and the decision to pursue a life of green shakes and weightlifting. The impact that our social, cultural and political world has on our health is as strong, if not stronger than the very DNA that makes up our individual bodies. We ignore the social context of health in medicine at our absolute peril. However, if these non-clinical factors of health are embraced in the practice of medicine, what we will see is a better way of caring, a more holistic approach to understanding patients that allows healthcare professionals like you to develop true pathways to health—supportive treatments that begin by speaking to the underlying causes of your patient's ill health. Finally, it is crucial to understand the social context of health because that is the context within which your patients' beliefs about health are formed. Luckily, that just so happens to be the subject of the next chapter.

Test Yourself

Throughout this book there will be opportunities to test your knowledge on what you have learnt. These have been written in the style of examination most commonly used in healthcare professional degrees so that you can use them as a way to study. Answers are available at the end of the book.

1. Identify the main difference between the behavioural-cultural and the materialist explanations.
2. A 7-year-old child is diagnosed with asthma. He lives in a deprived area of Birmingham where air pollution is high and the quality of housing is poor. This relationship between socio-economic status and health is referred to as:
    (a) Bad luck
    (b) Health inequalities
    (c) Socialism
    (d) Social selection

3. Provide a definition for the commercial determinants of health.
4. How does the inverse care law negatively affect health?
5. What are the three foci of the WHO definition of health?

Notes

1 In case you are thinking, 'fine, I'll work in a hospital', it is not much better. In deprived areas, hospital doctors shoulder heavier caseloads with fewer staff and equipment and more obsolete buildings and suffer recurrent crises around the availability of beds and replacement staff.

2 In case Adams is horrified by my take, here is their more academic way of putting it: 'we cannot explain socioeconomic inequalities in unhealthy body weight as due to differences in gluttony and laziness, nor view the solution as one of greater personal restraint and discipline'.

3 It is no coincidence that the TV drama series *Dopesick* chose Appalachia as the fictional home of its main characters. It is the very real home of stories that are likely very similar to the narrative told in the series.

4 Throughout this book, I will mostly use the term 'ethnic background', as it includes the widest group of people (e.g. ethnicity includes travellers, a recognised ethnicity) outside the 'white British' group used by the Office for National Statistics to characterise the majority of people living in the United Kingdom. However, even 'white British' is incomplete because not only is 'white' not a 'default normal' ethnicity, but of course there are 'white Australians', 'white Canadians' and lots of other 'white' groups who live in the United Kingdom. Despite this, most health data collected on ethnicity uses the 'white British' category. I'm not saying that's right—I'm just pointing out how we are constrained by the systems that collect the data we use in research. To help with this, where relevant to the data and argument, I will be more specific and use the term 'people of colour' to include all groups who do not identify as 'white'. People of colour will have experienced different issues and discrimination, then for example travellers or people from a white European background, and it is important to discuss this as it also impacts on their health individually and as a community.

5 Incidentally, there are whole books written on which mouse to use in science. For example, Suckow et al. (2023), which happens to be in its THIRD edition. We care more about using the right mice than about being inclusive of literally half the human population of the earth. Moreover, male lab mice remain the preference in research (Bailey, 2023).

References

Adams, J. (2020). 'Addressing socioeconomic inequalities in obesity: Democratising access to resources for achieving and maintaining a healthy weight.' *PLoS Medicine* 17(7): e1003243. https://doi.org/10.1371/journal.pmed.1003243

Albright, D.L., Johnson, K., Laha-Walsh, K., McDaniel, J. and McIntosh, S. (2021). 'Social determinants of opioid use among patients in rural primary care settings.' *Social Work in Public Health* 36(6): 723–731. https://doi.org/10.1080/19371918.2021.1939831

Amos, O. (2017). 'Why opioids are such an American problem.' *BBC News*, 25th October. Available at: https://www.bbc.com/news/world-us-canada-41701718

Appalachian Regional Commission (2011). *Economic overview of Appalachia—2011*. Available at: https://www.arc.gov/wp-content/uploads/2020/06/EconomicOverviewSept2011.pdf

Appalachian Regional Commission (2019). *Health disparities related to opioid misuse in Appalachia*. Available at: https://www.arc.gov/wp-content/uploads/2020/06/HealthDisparitiesRelatedto OpioidMisuseinAppalachiaApr2019.pdf

Bailey, S. (2023). 'Science experiments traditionally only used male mice—here's why that's a problem for women's health.' *The Conversation*, 15th August. Available at: https://theconversation.com/science-experiments-traditionally-only-used-male-mice-heres-why-thats-a-problem-for-womens-health-205963

Barr, H.L., Britton, J., Smyth, A.R. and Fogarty, A.W. (2011). 'Association between socioeconomic status, sex, and age at death from cystic fibrosis in England and Wales (1959 to 2008): Cross sectional study.' *British Medical Journal* 343: d4662. https://doi.org/10.1136/bmj.d4662

Beery, A.K. and Zucker, I. (2011.) 'Sex bias in neuroscience and biomedical research.' *Neuroscience & Biobehavioral Reviews* 35(3): 565–572. https://doi.org/10.1016/j.neubiorev.2010.07.002

Bell, R. (2017). *Psychosocial pathways and health outcomes: Informing action on health inequalities.* Institute of Health Equity. Available at: https://www.instituteofhealthequity.org/resources-reports/psychosocial-pathways-and-health-outcomes-informing-action-on-health-inequalities/psychosocial-pathways-and-health-outcomes.pdf

Benoit, C., Jeffery, A., Cleary, S., Masood, A., Paton, A. and Burt, C. (2023). *Health inequalities in Birmingham: Barriers encountered in underserved wards in East and West Birmingham.* Available at: https://research.aston.ac.uk/en/publications/health-inequalities-in-birmingham-barriers-encountered-in-underse

Blane, D., Smith, G.D. and Bartley, M. (1993). 'Social selection: What does it contribute to social class differences in health?' *Sociology of Health & Illness* 15: 1–15. https://doi.org/10.1111/j.1467-9566.1993.tb00328.x

Bodkin, H. and Horton, H. (2018). 'Cancer research toned down obesity campaign after "fat-shaming" backlash.' *The Telegraph*, 23rd March. Available at: https://www.telegraph.co.uk/news/2018/03/23/cancer-research-toned-obesity-campaign-fat-shaming-backlash/

British Heart Foundation (n.d.). *South Asian background.* Available at: https://www.bhf.org.uk/informationsupport/risk-factors/ethnicity/south-asian-background [accessed 21st April 2020].

Carey, G., Crammond, B. and De Leeuw, E. (2015). 'Towards health equity: A framework for the application of proportionate universalism.' *International Journal for Equity in Health* 14(1): 1–8. https://doi.org/10.1186/s12939-015-0207-6

Congressional Budget Office (2022). *The opioid crisis and recent federal policy responses.* Available at: https://www.cbo.gov/system/files/2022-09/58221-opioid-crisis.pdf

Cookson, R., Doran, T., Asaria, M., Gupta, I. and Mujica, F.P. (2021). 'The inverse care law re-examined: A global perspective.' *The Lancet* 397(10276): 828–838. https://doi.org/10.1016/S0140-6736(21)00243-9

Cornell Law School (n.d.). *At-will employment.* Available at: https://www.law.cornell.edu/wex/at-will_employment

Costello, E.J., Compton, S.N., Keeler, G. and Angoid, A. (2003). 'Relationships between poverty and psychopathology.' *Journal of the American Medical Association* 290: 2023–2029. https://doi.org/10.1001/jama.290.15.2023

Crenshaw, K. (1989). 'Demarginalizing the intersection of race and sex: A Black feminist critique of antidiscrimination doctrine, feminist theory and antiracist politics.' *University of Chicago Legal Forum* 1989(1): article 8. Available at: https://chicagounbound.uchicago.edu/cgi/viewcontent.cgi?article=1052&context=uclf

Criado Pérez, C. (2019). *Invisible women.* London: Chatto & Windus.

Dahlgren, G. and Whitehead, M. (1991). 'Policies and strategies to promote social equity in health. Background document to WHO—Strategy paper for Europe.' *Arbetsrapport* 2007: 14. Institute for Futures Studies.

Daugherty Biddison, E.L., Faden, R., Gwon, H.S., Mareiniss, D.P., Regenberg, A.C., Schoch-Spana, M., Schwartz, J. and Toner, E.S. (2019). 'Too many patients . . . A framework to guide statewide allocation of scarce mechanical ventilation during disasters.' *Chest* 155(4): 848–854. https://doi.org/10.1016/j.chest.2018.09.025

Feminist Rewrites (2018). *Feminist rewrites.* Available at: https://x.com/feministrewrite [accessed 15th August 2024].

Fisher, R. (2021). *'Levelling up' general practice in England: What should government prioritise?* The Health Foundation. Available at: www.health.org.uk/publications/long-reads/levelling-up-general-practice-in-england

Fisher, R., Allen, L., Malhotra, A.M. and Alderwick, H. (2022). *Tackling the inverse care law: Analysis of policies to improve general practice in deprived areas since 1990.* The Health Foundation. https://doi.org/10.37829/HF-2022-P09

Fox, M. (2023). 'Despite decades of promises, health research still overlooks women.' *The Guardian*, 20th November. Available at: https://www.theguardian.com/science/2023/nov/20/women-health-research-jill-biden-white-house

Garber, J. (2019). 'The culture that drives medication overload.' *Lown Institute*, 26th April. Available at: https://lowninstitute.org/the-culture-that-drives-medication-overload/

Gilmore, A.B., Fabbri, A., Baum, F., Bertscher, A., Bondy, K., Chang, H.J., Demaio, S., Erzse, A., Freudenberg, N., Friel, S., Hofman, K.J., Johns, P., Abdool Karim, S., Lacy-Nichols, J., de Carvalho, C.M.P., Marten, R., McKee, M., Petticrew, M., Robertson, L., Tangcharoensathien, V. and Thow, A.M. (2023). 'Defining and conceptualising the commercial determinants of health.' *The Lancet* 401(10383): 1194–1213. https://doi.org/10.1016/S0140-6736(23)00013-2

Government Accountability Office (2003). *Prescription drugs: OxyContin abuse and diversion and efforts to address the problem.* Publication GAO-04–110. Washington, DC: General Accounting Office. Available at: https://www.gao.gov/assets/gao-04-110.pdf

Hammes, S.R. (2024). 'Letter to Carolyn M. Mazure, 9th January.' *Endocrine Society.* Available at: https://www.endocrine.org/-/media/endocrine/files/advocacy/society-letters/2024/january/endocrine-society-response-to-whi-womens-health-rfi.pdf

The Health Foundation (n.d.). *'Black report' on health inequalities.* Available at: https://navigator.health.org.uk/theme/black-report-health-inequalities

Healy, B. (1991). 'The Yentl syndrome.' *The New England Journal of Medicine* 325: 274–276. https://doi.org/10.1056/NEJM199107253250408

Højsted, J. and Sjøgren, P. (2007). 'Addiction to opioids in chronic pain patients: A literature review.' *European Journal of Pain* 11(5): 490–518. https://doi.org/10.1016/j.ejpain.2006.08.004

Institute of Health Equity (2024). *Health inequalities, lives cut short.* Available at: https://www.instituteofhealthequity.org/in-the-news/press-releases-and-briefings-/health-inequalities-lives-cut-short

Kessler, A., Cohen, E. and Grise, K. (2018). 'The more opioids doctors prescribe, the more money they make.' *CNN*, 12th March. Available at: https://edition.cnn.com/2018/03/11/health/prescription-opioid-payments-eprise/index.html

King, S. (2021). 'Why are people of colour disproportionately impacted by the housing crisis?' *Shelter*, 5th February. Available at: https://blog.shelter.org.uk/why-are-people-of-colour-disproportionately-impacted-by-the-housing-crisis/

Krieger, N., Rehkopf, D.H., Chen, J.T., Waterman, P.D., Marcelli, E. and Kennedy, M. (2008). 'The fall and rise of US inequities in premature mortality: 1960–2002.' *PLoS Medicine* 5: e46. https://doi.org/10.1371/journal.pmed.0050046#

Leiwant, S., Weston Williamson, M. and Kashen, J. (2019). 'Brief 3: Inclusive paid sick time laws & the nonstandard workforce.' *Constructing 21st Century Rights for a Changing Workforce: A Policy Brief Series.* A Better Balance: The Work and Family Legal Center. Available at: https://www.abetterbalance.org/wp-content/uploads/2019/02/ABB_Policy-Brief-3.pdf

Levy, B., Paulozzi, L., Mack, K.A. and Jones, C.M. (2015). 'Trends in opioid analgesic-prescribing rates by specialty, U.S., 2007–2012.' *American Journal of Preventive Medicine* 49(3): 409–413. https://doi.org/10.1016/j.amepre.2015.02.020

Marmot, M., Allen, J., Boyce, T., Goldblatt, P. and Morrison, J. (2020). *Health equity in England: The Marmot review 10 years on.* Available at: https://www.instituteofhealthequity.org/resources-reports/marmot-review-10-years-on/the-marmot-review-10-years-on-full-report.pdf

Marmot, M., Allen, J., Goldblatt, P., Boyce, T., McNeish, D., Grady, M. and Geddes, I. (2010). *Fair society, healthy lives.* Available at: https://www.instituteofhealthequity.org/resources-reports/fair-society-healthy-lives-the-marmot-review/fair-society-healthy-lives-full-report-pdf.pdf

Marmot, M. and Wilkinson, R.G. (2001). 'Psychosocial and material pathways in the relation between income and health: A response to Lynch et al.' *British Medical Journal* 322(7296): 1233–1236. https://doi.org/10.1136/bmj.322.7296.1233

McCartney, G., Collins, C. and Mackenzie, M. (2013). 'What (or who) causes health inequalities: Theories, evidence and implications?' *Health Policy* 113(3): 221–227. https://doi.org/10.1016/j.healthpol.2013.05.021

Meier, B. (2003). *Pain killer*. Emmaus, PA: Rodale Press.

Merone, L., Tsey, K., Russell, D. and Nagle, C. (2022). 'Sex inequalities in medical research: A systematic scoping review of the literature.' *Women's Health Reports (New Rochelle)* 3(1): 49–59. https://doi.org/10.1089/whr.2021.0083

Moisi, E. (2020). 'Why a safe and stable home is crucial for people getting and keeping a job.' *The Crisis Blog*, 4th December. Available at: https://www.crisis.org.uk/about-us/the-crisis-blog/why-a-safe-and-stable-home-is-crucial-for-people-getting-and-keeping-a-job/ [accessed 12th August 2024].

Moody, L.N., Satterwhite, E. and Bickel, W.K. (2017). 'Substance use in rural Central Appalachia: Current status and treatment considerations.' *Journal of Rural Mental Health* 41(2): 123. https://doi.org/10.1037/rmh0000064

National Drug Intelligence Center (2001). *OxyContin diversion and abuse*. Available at: https://www.justice.gov/archive/ndic/pubs/651/index.htm

NHS England (2019). *Health survey for England 2018*. Available at: https://digital.nhs.uk/data-and-information/publications/statistical/health-survey-for-england/2018/summary [accessed 9th August 2024].

NHS England (2023). *NHS Workforce Race Equality Standard (WRES) 2022 data analysis report for NHS trusts*. Available at: https://www.england.nhs.uk/publication/nhs-workforce-race-equality-standard-2022/ [accessed 15th August 2024].

NHS England (n.d.a). *What are healthcare inequalities?* Available at: https://www.england.nhs.uk/about/equality/equality-hub/national-healthcare-inequalities-improvement-programme/what-are-healthcare-inequalities

NHS England (n.d.b). *Opioid prescribing for chronic pain*. Available at: https://www.england.nhs.uk/south/info-professional/safe-use-of-controlled-drugs/opioids/

NICE (2020). *COVID-19 rapid guideline: critical care in adults*. NICE Guideline [NG159]. Available at: https://www.nice.org.uk/guidance/ng159/resources [accessed 28th April 2020].

Nicholson, H.L. (2020). 'Socioeconomic status, fundamental cause theory, and prescription opioid use behaviors: A theoretical examination.' *Sociological Spectrum* 40(1): 1–32. https://doi.org/10.1080/02732173.2019.1707138

OECD (2020). *Post-education labour market outcomes*. Available at: https://www.oecd.org/en/topics/post-education-labour-market-outcomes.html

Office for National Statistics (2024). *National life tables—life expectancy in the UK: 2020 to 2022*. Available at: https://www.ons.gov.uk/peoplepopulationandcommunity/birthsdeathsandmarriages/lifeexpectancies/bulletins/nationallifetablesunitedkingdom/2020to2022

Paton, A. (2022). 'Fair is fair, right? Not when it comes to health.' *International Journal of Feminist Approaches to Bioethics* 5(1): 141–142. https://doi.org/10.3138/ijfab-15.1.20

Paton, A., Fooks, G., Maestri, G. and Lowe, P. (2020). *Submission of evidence on the disproportionate impact of COVID 19, and the UK government response, on ethnic minorities and women in the UK*. Available at: https://publications.aston.ac.uk/id/eprint/41460/1/Submission_of_evidence_for_Select_Committee_Aston_University_pdf.pdf

Patwardhan, V., Gil, G.F., Arrieta, A., Cagney, J., DeGraw, E. and Herbert, M.E. (2024). 'Differences across the lifespan between females and males in the top 20 causes of disease burden globally: A systematic analysis of the Global Burden of Disease Study 2021.' *The Lancet Public Health* 9: e282–94. Available at: https://www.thelancet.com/journals/lanpub/article/PIIS2468-2667(24)00053-7/fulltext

Purdue Pharma. (2001). *OxyContin marketing plan*. Stamford, CN: Purdue Pharma.

Rajput, V., Mookerjee, A.L. and Cagande, C. (2017). 'The contemporary hidden curriculum in medical education.' *MedEdPublish* 6: 1–13. Available at: https://mededpublish.org/articles/6-155

Raleigh, V. (2024). 'What is happening to life expectancy in England?' *The King's Fund*, 10th April. Available at: https://www.kingsfund.org.uk/insight-and-analysis/long-reads/whats-happening-life-expectancy-england

Ray, K. (2023). 'Racism and health equity.' *The Hastings Center for Bioethics*, 30th August. Available at: https://www.thehastingscenter.org/briefingbook/racism-and-health-equity/

Routen, A., Lekas, H., Harrison, J. and Khunti, K. (2023). 'Intersectionality in health equity research.' *British Medical Journal* 383: 2953. https://doi.org/10.1136/bmj.p2953

Royal College of Anaesthetists (n.d.). *Opioids aware*. Available at: https://fpm.ac.uk/opioids-aware

Shelter (n.d.). *The fight for home is a fight against racism*. Available at: https://england.shelter.org.uk/the_fight_for_home_is_a_fight_against_racism

Socialist Health Association (2012). *Inequalities in health: Report of a research working group* [cover image]. Available at: https://sochealth.co.uk/wp-content/uploads/2012/03/blackover.jpg [accessed 9th August 2024].

Socialist Health Association (n.d.). *Black report 6 explanation of health inequalities*. Available at: https://sochealth.co.uk/national-health-service/public-health-and-wellbeing/poverty-and-inequality/the-black-report-1980/black-report-6-explanation-of-health-inequalities/

SOPHIE Project (n.d.). *Conclusions*. Available at: http://www.sophie-project.eu/pdf/conclusions.pdf [accessed 16th August 2024].

Suckow, M.A., Hashway, S. and Pritchett-Corning, K. (2023). *The laboratory mouse*. Boca Raton: CRC Press. https://doi.org/10.1201/9780429353086

Taylor, L. (2018). 'Housing and health: An overview of the literature.' *Health Affairs*, 7th June. Available at: https://www.healthaffairs.org/content/briefs/housing-and-health-overview-literature

Thomas, B., Dorling, D. and Smith, G.D. (2010). 'Inequalities in premature mortality in Britain: Observational study from 1921 to 2007.' *British Medical Journal* 341: c3639. http://dx.doi.org/10.1136/bmj.c3639

Tudor Hart, J. (1971). 'The inverse care law.' *The Lancet* 297(7696): 405–412. Available at: https://www.thelancet.com/journals/lancet/article/PIIS0140–6736(71)92410-X/fulltext

US Department of Labor (2019). 'Private industry workers with sick leave benefits received 8 days per year at 20 years of service.' *The Economics Daily*. Available at: https://www.bls.gov/opub/ted/2019/private-industry-workers-with-sick-leave-benefits-received-8-days-per-year-at-20-years-of-service.htm

US Department of Labor (2022). 'Appalachian employment lagged rest of United States from 2001 to 2021.' *The Economics Daily*. Available at: https://www.bls.gov/opub/ted/2022/appalachian-employment-lagged-rest-of-united-states-from-2001-to–2021.htm [accessed 12th August 2024].

US Department of Labor (2023). *National compensation survey: Employee benefits in the United States, March 2023*. US Bureau of Labor Statistics. Available at: https://www.bls.gov/ncs/ebs/benefits/2023/home.htm

US Department of Labor (n.d.). *Sick leave*. Available at: https://www.dol.gov/general/topic/workhours/sickleave#:~:text=Currently%2C%20there%20are%20no%20federal,does%20require%20unpaid%20sick%20leave

US Food and Drug Administration (2015). *Prescription drug advertising | Questions and answers*. Available at: https://www.fda.gov/drugs/prescription-drug-advertising/prescription-drug-advertising-questions-and-answers

Van Zee, A. (2009). 'The promotion and marketing of oxycontin: Commercial triumph, public health tragedy.' *American Journal of Public Health* 99(2): 221–227. Available at: https://www.ncbi.nlm.nih.gov/pmc/articles/PMC2622774/pdf/221.pdf

Vlassoff, C. (2007). 'Gender differences in determinants and consequences of health and illness.' *Journal of Health, Population and Nutrition* 25(1): 47–61. Available at: https://pmc.ncbi.nlm.nih.gov/articles/PMC3013263/

Vowles, K.E., McEntee, M.L., Julnes, P.S., Frohe, T., Ney, J.P. and van der Goes, D.N. (2015). 'Rates of opioid misuse, abuse, and addiction in chronic pain: A systematic review and data synthesis.' *Pain* 156: 569–576. https://doi.org/10.1097/01.j.pain.0000460357.01998.f1

Weston Williamson, M. (2024). 'The state of paid sick time in the U.S. in 2024.' *Center for American Progress*, 17th January. Available at: https://www.americanprogress.org/article/the-state-of-paid-sick-time-in-the-u-s-in-2024/

Wilkinson, R.G. (1990). 'Income distribution and mortality: A "natural" experiment.' *Sociology of Health & Illness* 12: 391–412. https://doi.org/10.1111/1467-9566.ep11340405

Woodard, C. (2023). 'America's surprising partisan divide on life expectancy.' *Politico*, 1st September. Available at: https://www.politico.com/news/magazine/2023/09/01/america-life-expectancy-regions-00113369

World Health Organisation (2008). *Closing the gap in a generation: Health equity through action on the social determinants of health. Final Report of the Commission on Social Determinants of Health.* Geneva: World Health Organization. Available at: https://www.who.int/publications/i/item/WHO-IER-CSDH-08.1

World Health Organisation (2018). *WHO housing and health guidelines.* Available at: https://www.who.int/publications/i/item/9789241550376

World Health Organisation (2023). *Commercial determinants of health.* Available at: https://www.who.int/news-room/fact-sheets/detail/commercial-determinants-of-health

How people understand their health

In the first chapter, I asked you to consider the question 'what is health'? For your patients, the answer to this question will be varied. They will understand health as relative to their own lives and will make decisions about their health based on that understanding. This understanding will not always match yours; the information that people use to construct their beliefs about health are unique to them. Most of the time there is a shared belief, but increasingly there is not (we will discuss that shortly) and it can be helpful to understand how health beliefs are developed so that you can better communicate with your patients about their health needs in ways that fit their understandings of their own health.

Perceptions of health

There have been many attempts to categorise health over the years. The WHO definition remains the go-to for the general concept of health, but how do individuals themselves understand their health? This, to my mind, is impossible to answer in a satisfactory way, as most people have unique views on health that do not fit neatly into categories. Life is messy, the lives we live are messy and we make decisions about our health in messy ways. However, there have been attempts to develop concepts or perceptions of health over the years. It is useful to look at some of these categorisations, as it shows us that society itself wants to make sense of the way we understand health.

Sartorius (2006) describes three ways of perceiving health that can help us to think more about different understandings of 'health'. Though Sartorius does not name these three ways, over time this description has developed into an understanding of health as positive, negative and functional. A positive perception of health is one where the individual attends to their overall wellbeing, seeking an equilibrium in their lives that allows them to live the healthiest version of that life every day (Bodryzlova and Moullec, 2023; Sartorius, 2006). The positive perception of health draws heavily on the WHO definition of health, where health involves more than simply not being ill.

DOI: 10.4324/9781032677552-3

Some argue that this means people with a positive understanding of their health try every day to be the healthiest they can be and that they prioritise health, though this remains highly contested, with no one definition being agreed upon or most prominent (Bodryzlova and Moullec, 2023).

A negative perception of health is where health is understood as the absence of disease or illness. No other dimensions of health are relevant. Someone is either ill with a recognised disease and thus 'unhealthy' or they are free of illness and thus 'healthy' (Krahn et al., 2021; Sartorius, 2006). There are some obvious limitations to this particular way of conceptualising health. First, it puts the individual at the whims (if not the mercy) of the medical paradigm. This means that 'medicine', that is someone's doctor, decides if they are healthy or not, regardless of how they feel. With changing trends in medicine, this also means that a person could find themself classified as 'unhealthy' one day by medicine and 'healthy' the next (Sartorius, 2006). There are several instances of this happening over time that illustrate the absurdity of allowing health to be dictated solely by the paradigm of medicine. For example, the following have, at various points in the history of medicine, been considered 'illness': homosexuality (a mental disorder until 1987); being a woman with almost any ailment (known as hysteria, again a mental disorder until the 1980s); and enjoying sex (nymphomania, a uniquely female 'disease' that somehow never afflicted men). It is worth noting here that what medicine considers a disease can often mirror the views of society at the time. Homosexuality was viewed as abhorrent for centuries in British society. In fact, it remained illegal in various forms and institutions in the United Kingdom until 2017, when legislation that allowed the sacking of homosexual individuals in the Merchant Navy was finally repealed (Tatchell, 2017). Hysteria no longer exists as a diagnosis; it is now widely accepted that it was used as a 'catch-all' term for the unique health issues faced by women, allowing these to be dismissed as in the mind of the patient. Nymphomania reflected a societal view, held for hundreds if not thousands of years, that sex really should not be something that women want to 'do'. Thus, as the last two chapters have shown, it is not always possible to trust that medicine has our best interests at heart.

Viewing health solely as the absence of disease also causes trouble for people who do not neatly fit into the idea that disease can be 'cured' and thus rendered absent. As we have already seen with the biomedical model of disease, chronic illness sufferers do not fit into this paradigm. Chronic illness can come and go and change in severity, meaning that sometimes people feel ill with it and their symptoms 'classically' indicate they are ill, and sometimes they do not. I will further discuss chronic illness shortly, but the point here is that, as the WHO, the biopsychosocial model and this book are showing you, a person's health is usually more complex than whether they have a cold (and the expected textbook symptoms) or not.

Finally, many people will have a functional understanding of health, where they consider themselves healthy if they can basically carry on life as usual. Sartorius (2006) says that this implies an absence of disease or impairment, but the functional definition used currently is less specific. 'As usual' means many different things to different people. The International Classification of Functioning, Disability and Health (known as the ICF) takes a more contextual approach, viewing functional health as a balance between the body someone lives in and the world they live in with that body

(World Health Organisation, 2001). If those interactions are positive or neutral, then 'health' is achieved. Should they be negative, the ICF views it as 'disability' (World Health Organisation, 2001). The ICF is an example of the biopsychosocial framework in action, giving us an example of what that framework can look like when applied to policy and practice (Leonardi et al., 2022). It is by no means perfect and is often criticised and disputed, though it is interesting that the ICF has been responsive to change over time, indicating a willingness to grow and learn in a changing environment (Sykes et al., 2021; World Health Organisation, 2018).

Lay beliefs and lay epidemiology

What people believe about their health changes over time in general but also over their own lifetimes. Think back to the last time you got ill. You likely had an understanding and narrative for how and why it happened. It will be specific to you. In addition to being the normal way that people make sense of the world around them, this reasoning for why a person is ill is called lay epidemiology. Lay epidemiology is the way a person understands why and how illness happens, and why it happens to a particular person at a particular time. We commonly observe and generate hypotheses from the experiences of those around us, and health is no different. For example, with two young children, my usual go-to for understanding whatever lurgy I have at any given time is to assume I have picked it up from either nursery or school—known and proven incubators for germs and illness (Godoy, 2023). Being a parent is thus a critical part of my own understanding of my own health. It influences the way I make decisions about my health, including behaviours around medication and taking time off from work. These are some of my lay beliefs about health.

Lay beliefs about health are how people understand and make sense of health and illness. They are most often constructed by people with no specialist knowledge, though healthcare professionals hold lay beliefs about health just like everyone else. It is a misnomer to assume that lay beliefs are just watered-down or even incorrect medical knowledge. They are much more complex than that. Lay beliefs are not really even 'lay' or 'amateur', given that they are constructed to match the understanding that individuals have about their own lives—an area in which they are by necessity experts (Paton et al., 2020). It must be acknowledged that there can be gaps between lay concepts of health and the relevant medical knowledge about those concepts. However, it would be foolish, and dangerous for patients, for healthcare professionals to assume that these gaps mean they can ignore lay beliefs. As with so many aspects of health, lay beliefs are socially constructed and socially embedded (Sensky, 1996). Different communities, cultures and countries will influence an individual's lay beliefs about health. As people can move between communities, cultures and countries, lay beliefs also have the potential to change and are often not fixed throughout a person's lifetime. This can lead some to argue that lay beliefs are thus irrelevant, but they are not. Make no mistake—lay beliefs are real beliefs that impact on health behaviours and the decisions people make about their health (Paton et al., 2020). They are complex and drawn from various creditable and non-creditable sources, and while that creditability is not always an accepted clinical source, it is a key source to the patient (Paton et al., 2020). Frustrating as it may be to healthcare professionals, people make decisions about their health that are not solely based on best clinical practice. Even more importantly (and equally frustrating for you, their healthcare provider), this does not mean they have made the wrong decision about their health either (Paton et al., 2020).

The lay referral system

It is not just a person's own beliefs that influence their decisions. Over a two-week period, about 75% of the population will experience one or more symptoms of ill health. This is pretty normal. Most people will not act on about half of the symptoms they experience. Thirty-five per cent of symptoms will result in some kind of lay care, usually over-the-counter medication such as cold medicine or pain relief. Twelve per cent of symptoms will lead to a consultation with a primary healthcare professional, usually a GP. This means that on any given day, most symptoms are never reported to a doctor. This is known as the symptom or illness iceberg (Elliott et al., 2011).

So how do people decide if they are going to act on symptoms? It is relatively rare for someone to decide to visit a doctor or pharmacist without first discussing their symptoms with others. Up to three-quarters of those visiting a doctor have discussed their symptoms with another person, which is called the lay referral system. The lay referral system is the chain of advice-seeking contacts that the sick make with other lay people prior to—or instead of—seeking help from healthcare professionals. The 'instead of' clause of that definition is really quite important. As we know from the symptom iceberg, rightly or wrongly, many people will choose to ignore their symptoms or not seek help for them at all.

As a healthcare professional, understanding how the lay referral system works and why people use it is vital to understanding your patient when and if they do eventually show up in your clinic. It is often the reason why people might have delayed seeking help or used alternative medicines or services; it can also indicate how important (or not) your role as their healthcare professional is to their understanding of their own health. How, why and when people consult their doctor, for example, is just as important to your understanding of their health as what is wrong with their health in the first place. The lay referral system can illuminate the reasoning behind these choices, which in turn will also help you understand the extent to which patients will use the recommended health services and medication they need.

In fact, patients fall into three broad categories when it comes to the way health beliefs influence health behaviours: 'deniers and distancers', 'accepters' and 'pragmatists' (Adams et al., 1997). Let's unpack these terms for a better understanding of how crucial health beliefs are in influencing behaviour.

Deniers and distancers

Deniers deny they have an illness. Even when faced with a diagnosis, they will not accept that diagnosis. Distancers are slightly different. Distancers will deny the degree of illness they have. For example, they will agree with a diagnosis of asthma, but they will say that they do not have 'proper' asthma. That they are just a bit 'chesty'. Normally, deniers and distancers act in these ways because they believe their symptoms do not interfere with everyday life. Using the language from earlier in the chapter, they have a functional definition of health. What does this mean for their healthcare providers? Well, deniers and distancers can use complex or drastic strategies to hide illness from others. They will be unlikely to seek help and when they do, they will be unwilling to comply with the recommended treatment. This is because taking medication relies on accepting their illness identity—and they do not. Using our example of asthma, deniers and distancers will not use inhalers or attend asthma clinics because they believe they either do not have asthma or are 'just a bit chesty'. As we will shortly see, this is often because of the stigma or shame that having an illness causes in their society. Either way, the outcome for their health is the same: they do not receive the treatment they need for their illness.

Accepters

Accepters are your dream patient as a healthcare professional. They do what it says on the tin: they accept their diagnosis and follow their health professionals' advice completely. They are also happy to accept the impact that the diagnosis has on their understanding of their own health. As a result, they view a 'normal life' as one where they control their symptoms by taking the recommended treatment or medication. In the case of our asthma example, they accept their asthma diagnosis and have no issues complying with treatment. They see no shame in having asthma and no stigma in using an inhaler in public because of that asthma.

Pragmatists

Pragmatists walk the line between deniers, distancers and accepters. They acknowledge their diagnosis, and they are willing to use some preventive medication or treatment, but only when they feel the illness is bad. Again, shame and stigma likely come into play in the pragmatist's approach to their health. In the case of asthma, they will meet their healthcare professional halfway. They may accept the diagnosis of asthma, but will view it as a mild illness that only requires treatment such as an inhaler when they consider themselves to be having an acute asthma attack. What they consider acute and what is clinically acute may differ dramatically, but the pragmatist uses their own measures to guide their health actions.

Health literacy

Health literacy brings all the above concepts together. This is not about the ability of a patient to read a pamphlet or understand the instructions on over-the-counter medication. Health literacy is a complex set of actions whereby people are able to access the information they need about their health, understand that information and then use it to make decisions about promoting and maintaining their good health (Nutbeam, 1998). As such, this literacy is both an individual and public good. It is also a vital component of good health, and so despite the individualistic nature of its definition, population-level health literacy is increasingly seen as a goal to improve health outcomes regionally, nationally and globally (Rudd, 2015). People with higher health literacy are more likely to act to improve their health and tend to have better access to healthcare. In fact, improved health literacy is strongly linked to improved universal healthcare coverage. As a result, health literacy reduces social determinants such as poverty by reducing and protecting against the risk of catastrophic health events that can impoverish individuals, families and communities (World Health Organisation, n.d.). Improving health literacy is also a way to mitigate against and even reduce the health inequalities that exist within societies and globally.

Stigma and shame in health

However, health literacy and health beliefs are strongly shaped by society, just like every aspect of health. This can of course have negative consequences. Two of the strongest negative influences on health beliefs are stigma and shame. They exist at some level in all of health and healthcare, but are very keenly experienced within the world of chronic and long-term illness, so that is a good case study for exploring the influence that stigma and shame have on health. Let's start by gaining a better understanding of what chronic and long-term illness are, before applying the concepts of stigma and shame.

Chronic and long-term illness

A chronic or long-term illness cannot be cured by medicine, only controlled with medicine and/or other treatments and therapies. You will see both terms used, but I consider them to be interchangeable, as their definitions are the same. I prefer to use chronic illness and will throughout this book. What is a key to chronic illness is that it normally never goes away. A person has a chronic illness for life and their life is different because of their diagnosis. Even if they can control many or all of the symptoms with medication or treatment of some kind, they are no longer the person they were before their diagnosis. The diagnosis and ongoing management of their illness alters them forever.

In the United Kingdom, about a quarter of the population has some kind of chronic illness. Chronic illness in the UK population is predicted to increase over time, including a person having more than one chronic illness at the same time. The NHS spends a significant amount of its time and money caring for people with chronic illness—about 70% of the overall NHS budget is spent on this every year (Nuffield Trust, 2025). How the NHS will cope moving forward with a growing population living with one or more chronic illnesses is one of the acknowledged major challenges for its future (Dunn et al., 2023).

Chronic illness not only impacts our health but also, directly and indirectly, our social interactions and our ability to perform our role in the world in which we live, whether that role be as a parent, spouse or friend. Modern sociological theory on chronic illness is derived from studies that examine these interactions in depth, focusing on the lived experiences of people with chronic illnesses managing and negotiating the effects of the illness on their everyday life. It is when unpacking these theories that we see how complex living with illness really is.

The experience of illness: a little bit of theory

Theories that explore the experience of illness are where the contrast between acute illness and chronic illness is at its sharpest. As we have seen in previous chapters, throughout history and within different societies, there have been beliefs about what sickness is and who sick people are. The sociological theories are no different, examining not just the experience of a 'sick' person but also what is expected of them. For a long time, the experience of illness was largely seen in two distinct ways: functional or interpretive. The functional understanding of illness experience is considered largely defunct in sociology, yet it is still taught in medicine, so we will briefly cover it below. There are now various interpretive ways of understanding illness experience. We are going to focus on a few that influence the way we understand the relationship between society, health and health beliefs and behaviours within medicine.

Bad medicine: understanding Parsons' 'sick role'

Talcott Parsons proposed the concept of the 'Sick Role' in his 1951 work, *Illness and the Role of the Physician: A Sociological Perspective*. It was the first concept in sociology that explicitly involved medical sociology and part of the 'functional' movement in the field. Parsons described the sick role as a temporary, medically sanctioned form of deviant behaviour. Society, as a general rule, does not like or tolerate deviance, but Parsons argued that being ill was an exception to this. So long as certain rules were followed, the deviance was 'allowed' by the society. These rules include: a sick person can be excused from their usual duties, and the sick person is expected to seek professional advice and to adhere to treatment so that they are cured and get better. The idea is that they can take temporary leave from society, but they need to step back in as soon as they are better. Their deviance is fleeting and cannot last long.

Additionally, a person will not be held responsible for their ill health and the consequences of that ill health, such as missing work, if they also adhere to the rules of seeking medical help and complying with medical advice. As a result, exceptions can be made for the ill person to step away from their usual responsibilities, so long as they are approved by a doctor. This was a big change. Remember that the idea of personal responsibility in health loomed large in the twentieth century and that in 1951, most countries did not yet have a health service that people could access for free. The concept of the 'sick role' was likely viewed as a bit of a saviour here, as being ill was no longer completely the fault of the patient. It also granted huge amounts of power to an already very powerful profession: doctors. Medical practitioners were now empowered to sanction the temporary absence of patients from the workforce and family duties, as well as absolve them of blame. Doctors could say when a patient was ill, which had (hopefully) positive consequences for their ability to get better.

The sick role was a product of its time, when medicine and doctors were all-powerful and ill health could easily ruin someone's whole life. However, as a concept in the modern world and in modern medicine, Parsons' sick role does not stand up to scrutiny. It is outdated and fails to account for the fundamental aspects of health and medicine that are so basic to us, and yet completely ignored by Parsons. Let's take a moment to look at the reasons why the sick role no longer works.

First, not all illnesses are temporary. You may have been wondering why we jumped from chronic illness to a defunct sociological theory by a white man, but I hope it now makes sense. Chronic illnesses cannot be cured. They are not temporary, but forever. People with chronic illness can therefore NEVER fulfil the sick role, as they can never get better. However, they are, by definition, sick. That someone with a chronic illness is ill is without question. Given that almost three-quarters of healthcare spending in the United Kingdom is spent on people with chronic illness, it is clear that the sick role simply does not apply to most people.

Relatedly, the sick role does not account for structural limits to a person's ability to 'be' ill. As the previous chapters have shown, not everybody has the luxury of being ill, sick role or not. For example, government support such as mandatory sick leave and pay is critical to whether a person can even assume the sick role to begin with. Where there is a lack of structural support via legislation and policy, there will be very ill people who cannot take a day off work, even if they want to. This leads us to another limitation of the role: it does not acknowledge differences between people, cultures or societies. Different cultures and societies will have different expectations, understandings and behaviours around illness and the idea of illness being 'deviant' may be a completely foreign concept.

Finally, the sick role does not acknowledge individual agency in defining and coping with illness. As we already know, both individually and within the societies where we live, we have different definitions of what counts as healthy and unhealthy. The sick role imposes a single way of understanding this on people and also a single way of dealing with ill health. As is characteristic of mid-twentieth-century medicine, the sick role gives all the power to the doctor and none to the patient. It should come as no surprise that medical ethics gained momentum as a discipline in the 1950s as a direct reaction to these power dynamics.

All of this is why, 73 years later, the sick role is woefully out of touch with the world in which the sick live and their experiences of living in that world. It continues to be taught in medicine despite widespread acknowledgment that it is not fit for purpose. I suspect this is because modern medicine was largely founded in those mid-twentieth-century years, and so the theories that defined beliefs around health have resulted in hangovers that continue to be perpetuated today. Additionally, the most senior members of medical staff in most countries were trained during those years, and many still carry those beliefs with them. My hope is that, in the next decade, we see the 'sick role' move from a live theory taught in medical schools to one discussed in history of medicine courses instead. If you attend my courses, you will know I only include it in the syllabus as an example of how even sociology can get things wrong.

Illness narratives

As medical sociology evolved, it became increasingly clear that the sick role could not account for patients' varied experiences of illness. Instead, it was more helpful to capture these experiences by listening to the stories of people with chronic illness; thus the interpretive illness narrative approach was developed (Bury and Monaghan, 2013).

Illness narratives are incredibly useful because examining them has brought to light the huge amount of implicit and explicit work, in varying forms, that people with chronic illness have to engage in every day. What I mean by 'work' is the everyday actions that people with chronic illness must perform just to live with and manage their illness. By listening to people's stories about living with chronic illness, it is possible to categorise these types of work, as seen below (Figure 3.1).

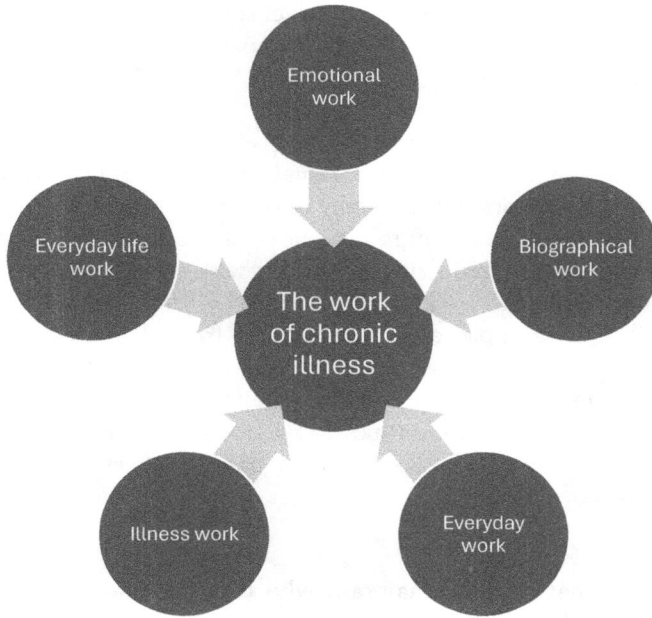

Figure 3.1 The Work of Chronic Illness.

Illness work

Illness work is work relating to the illness itself: things like getting a diagnosis and managing symptoms. However, sometimes they are not straightforward. People may have to fight to get a diagnosis, and even once they have one, they have to learn not only to manage the symptoms alongside a doctor but also to carry out self-management of that illness. Illness work is complex and can be negative for the patient, as they shoulder the burden alone. This makes them responsible for a condition that is outside of their control and very difficult and exhausting to manage themselves. You must remember that people with chronic illness are ill. There is conflicting evidence in this area; self-management (i.e. engaging in illness work) has been shown both to improve and to worsen the impact of chronic illness on a person (Liddy et al., 2014; Barker et al., 2018). As a result, it is not clear whether patients gain real agency, support or understanding from the many self-management programmes being pushed by most healthcare systems.

Everyday life work

Everyday life work involves people deploying coping mechanisms and strategies, both for themselves and those around them, to 'normalise' the illness itself within the person's life. It requires patients to bring together the medical work of treating their symptoms with the mental load of coping with their illness, so that they can manage their condition and its impact. An example of everyday life work is making decisions about the mobilisation of resources to manage the illness, such as balancing the demands on others caused by the illness, but also working out how to remain independent. It is a huge amount of work and effort whereby the chronically ill patient either tries very hard to maintain the person they were pre-diagnosis or has to come to terms with a whole new version of themselves.

Emotional work

Everyday work often spills over into emotional work. Emotional work is work that people do to protect the emotional wellbeing of others and themselves. When someone has a chronic illness, even just maintaining normal activities becomes a deliberately conscious act. It can be hard and tiring to interact with others, and, as a result, people with chronic illnesses have to spend more time and effort on the emotional relationships in their lives. For example, due to restrictions from their chronic illness, people may strategically withdraw or restrict their social activities. As a result, friendships may be disrupted, and keeping these friendships alive requires emotional work on the part of the person with the chronic illness. Emotional work may also involve downplaying pain or other symptoms and presenting a happier, cheerier version of oneself to protect the emotions of others.

Biographical work

With all that emotional work to maintain who they are and the relationships they have, it is no surprise that there are repercussions for the person in terms of their own understanding of themself. There is often a loss of self that is not well accounted for by non-narrative theories of illness. Effectively, the person they were, their self-image, crumbles away, but without an equally valued new version of themself developing to take its place (Charmaz, 1983). This can leave people with chronic illness struggling to figure out who they are now, in the new normal that is living with their illness. The result is biographical work, meaning the constant struggle experienced by a person with chronic illness when trying to lead a valued life and maintain a positive definition of their own self.

The transition from person-without-a-chronic-illness to person-with-a-chronic-illness has been described as 'biographical disruption' (Bury, 1982). Biographical disruption focuses on people's experience of the onset of illness as a disruptive event in their lives. It identifies three ways that the onset of illness changes how we understand ourselves, thus 'disrupting' our existing biography (Bury, 1982).

1. A disruption of everyday activities takes place. As a result of the onset of illness, everyday actions are no longer easy or even possible to carry out. There is a disruption of those things that we take for granted that we can do every day. This forces the person to focus more on their body than they did before the illness; they may even have to seek out extra support to do what they previously had been able to do themselves.
2. A rethinking of the self occurs. As we discussed with regards to biographical work, there has been a disruption in who the person understands themselves to be. They are no longer who they were before the onset of illness and they must now find a way to redefine who they are after.
3. The person has to mobilise their resources. These resources must be used to face, and live in, the new reality caused by the onset of illness. These can be financial,

emotional, social and physical resources that must be either redeployed or reviewed in some way to help meet the new needs of the person.

Biographical disruption is a useful way of understanding what illness can do to a person and their understanding of their own self. It acknowledges the differences between individuals and does not try to suggest that the experience of chronic illness is generic. That being said, it does have some limitations that are worth considering. First, and quite obviously, the concept of biographical disruption does not deal with conditions from birth. If someone is born with a chronic illness, there is no 'disruption' to their biography because they have always understood themself to be the way that they are. However, they will still engage in all the same work as people who develop chronic illness later in life. Furthermore, some social groups expect illness more than others, and so illness is not necessarily understood as a disruption to their selves—they were expecting it in some way. In this situation, the onset of illness is less of a disruption; it would be better described as biographical continuity or biographical flow (Faircloth et al., 2004). A good example of this is that older people may see chronic illness as biographically 'normal' and thus may not experience the same level of biographical disruption or engage in as much biographical work as younger people diagnosed with a chronic illness (Kirkpatrick et al., 2018).

Identity work
Of course, if a person's understanding of themselves is disrupted, then it is equally difficult for them to understand the new 'them'. Identity work is a person's process of reconstructing their self now that they have a chronic illness. It can be wide-ranging work, often across a spectrum, in that the person is fighting on multiple fronts. The reason why identity work is so hard to define is that different conditions have different consequences and result in different changes to a person's life. People are also very different. A chronic illness will affect the way people see themselves and the way others see them in different ways. However, there is a risk that the illness will become a defining feature of the person's identity, especially if there is significant change to their lives or stigma attached to their illness.

Stigma and mental health
Stigma shapes a significant amount of the work people with chronic illness must engage in, and more generally, is a key feature of health and medicine around the world. One category of chronic illness that is prevalent in most societies is mental illness. Mental health has become an increasingly important part of our understanding of overall good health. A quarter of people in England experience a mental health issue every year (Mind, 2020). To put this into context, based on the 2024 population, that is about 14.5 million people dealing with a mental health concern every single year (Office for National Statistics, n.d.). It is very likely you will treat several patients a day who have a mental health condition. More importantly for our purposes in this chapter, many of the common mental health conditions are also considered chronic.

Socially, mental health conditions are some of the most stigmatised conditions in health. What do I mean by this? Because we live in societies with other people, there is always some difference between our 'virtual social identity', meaning how we are understood by others, and our 'actual social identity', meaning the qualities we actually possess (Goffman, 1963, p. 2). People experience stigma, i.e. a negative attitude towards them from others, when there is a discrepancy between the two—people are perceived differently to the way they understand themselves to be. As a result of this discrepancy, the identity of the person is damaged in some way.

This damage occurs because within our social world, there exist accepted and unaccepted attributes. These may relate to the perceived or actual character of someone (for example being greedy or lazy) or their physical characteristics (for example a disfigurement of some kind). Rightly, or very often wrongly, each society will have embedded beliefs about the worth of people based on these characteristics. Stigma reduces the stigmatised person to a lesser member of a society by discrediting them within that society, thus taking them from being a 'whole person' in the eyes of the society to a 'tainted' and 'discounted' one (Goffman, 1963, p. 3). In other words, once stigmatised, the world around the person no longer views them as a real person with the same rights, needs, wants and wishes as 'normal' people. A stigmatised person is thus considered a lesser person and, as a result, can be, and is, treated differently.

Mental health has a long history of stigmatisation in most societies globally. In the United Kingdom alone, 90% of the people with some sort of mental health condition report feeling stigmatised or discriminated against because of their condition (Mental Health Foundation, 2021). As a result of the stigma around mental health, people with a chronic mental condition can struggle to function as they want to in society, as they may find themselves excluded from jobs they want or be unable to find appropriate housing, to provide just two examples (Mental Health Foundation, 2021). Mental health stigma stems largely from stereotypes that portray people with mental health conditions as dangerous, violent and unstable (Doll et al., 2022). The media is a particularly bad perpetrator; not only does it exaggerate the nature of people with a mental health condition, but it over-dramatises the fear, rejection and general discrimination of people with mental illness (Stuart, 2006; Wahl, 1995). The result is that people with a mental illness can experience different types of stigma, often all at once.

Types of stigma

Stigma can be experienced in different ways; this in turn influences the impact that it can have on a person. First, stigma can be discreditable or discredited. The difference between the two relates to whether the illness can be concealed or is easily apparent to others. Where discreditable stigma is experienced, it is because nothing can be seen, but the fear is that if the person's stigmatised trait is 'found out', then people will treat them differently. Depression and anxiety are examples of conditions with discreditable stigma. Discreditable stigma is an internal stigma, or what is sometimes described as intrapersonal or felt stigma: the person is aware of the stigma that surrounds their condition in society, has internalised this stigma in the form of shame and feels both shame about having the condition and fear that someone will find out (Corrigan et al., 2010). When people experience this type of discreditable, felt stigma, they act differently than they otherwise would want, as they expect discrimination should they be 'discovered' to have a condition (Gray, 2002). For example, people experiencing felt stigma may not seek the support they need for their condition or may withdraw from their social support circles for fear of being discovered.

Discredited stigma is the opposite. Here, the physically visible characteristics of the condition 'outs' the person; they cannot hide their condition, which leads to discrimination and judgement born from existing stigma—for example a physical disability. Also described as enacted or interpersonal stigma, this stigma normally manifests itself through unfair treatment of the person with the condition (Gray, 2002). Enacted stigma can stop people getting the social and financial support they need by limiting where they can work and live and even with whom they can be friends. Tourette's syndrome is a good example of this, as sufferers' tics mean that they cannot hide the condition (though Tourette's is actually classified as a neurological disorder, not a mental health illness, despite often being described as such) (Hermetet, n.d.).

This stigma spills out from everyday interactions between people to include systemic or structural stigma. Structural stigma is the stigma people experience from the institutions, laws and policies that exist in a society, which actively constrain a person's ability to access the resources and support they need for their own wellbeing (Hatzenbuehler and Link, 2014). A non-medical example of structural stigma is the segregation laws that existed in the United States. These laws prohibited people of colour from accessing certain parts of society and the associated resources that came with that access. Within medicine, mental illness is most impacted by structural stigma, which permeates through every level of medicine and allied healthcare, including healthcare training itself (Macfarlane et al., 2025).

The reason I have spent so long discussing mental health and mental illnesses in this section is that it is not just broader society where mental health stigma is an issue—it is especially prevalent in medicine itself. In medicine, the stigma against mental illness is so strong that it can prevent people from getting the help they actually need because their own healthcare professional has stigmatising ideas about that person's health, which impacts the way they treat the patient and the quality of care they provide (Knaak et al., 2017). Stigma can also 'layer' on to an individual; they can experience stigma relating to more than one thing at a time. For example, in the United Kingdom, Black people are four times as likely to be detained under the Mental Health Act and are arrested twice as often using section 136 (Mind, n.d.). It should come as no surprise that this group are less likely to seek and receive help. Furthermore, the help they do receive tends to be less useful and more forceful than that provided to white people experiencing the same mental health issues (Mind, n.d.). Further layered-on stigma can be based on gender, employment or ancestors' country of origin (Mind, n.d.). As we saw in chapter 2, racism is a key part of health, so it is unsurprising that it is also a key part of the way people experience stigma and shame relating to health.

Social media and health influencers: a perfect, misinformed storm

As the ways that we communicate and understand the world around us change, so do our health beliefs. In this final section, we bring several of the previously discussed concepts together to discuss the impact that social media has on health beliefs, as there are direct consequences for the health of your patient and the way you interact with them about their health. Social media use is widespread in most societies in the twenty-first century, especially in English-speaking countries. It will come as no surprise that as social media use has risen, there has been a steady increase in people turning to these platforms for health information and advice. A recent report found that 26% of millennials and 33% of Gen Z use social media for health information, with TikTok being the most popular platform (Ireland, n.d.). The generational divide is strong here, with only 5% of baby boomers doing the same (Ireland, n.d.). For patients with chronic illness, the numbers reveal a significant shift in where people are getting, and prefer to get, their health information these days. Thirty-eight per cent said they no longer used their doctors as regular sources of health information; instead, their preference was for online health influencers and social media (McQuater, 2023). Increasingly, online communities and support groups have become a key part of support for chronic illness. Information is traded there just as it is in the clinical setting.

The reasons for turning to social media are varied. For example, about half of respondents from the United Kingdom said they were frustrated with how little time they were able to spend with doctors. Globally, the move to social media and health influencers strongly relates to dissatisfaction with the current doctor-patient relationship. Patients feel unheard and discriminated against and often report a perceived lack of empathy from their doctors, all of which causes them to look elsewhere for their health information (Paton et al., 2020). In many ways, social media as a source of health information is part of a wider, decades-long trend that has seen the power of doctors as the 'keepers' of health information wane. For most people, this has coincided with a greater desire to understand their health and have more control over it. This is especially important for people with chronic illness, who are largely left on their own to self-manage their conditions. In many ways, this shift, which has seen sources of information about health arise outside of the healthcare environment, is an important part of facilitating that self-management and promoting and supporting patient autonomy (Paton et al., 2020).

For example, social media health campaigns can support health literacy whilst reducing stigma around certain conditions such as mental illness (Jafar et al., 2023). That being said, there is a big caveat to the use of social media and influencers as sources of health information—they, like almost all digital health sources, are unregulated in most of the world (Paton, 2022). This means that outside of a handful of government agencies, such as the NHS in the United Kingdom, there is no way for people accessing this information to know if the information provided is correct. This can lead people to come to incorrect conclusions about their own health and even to make decisions about their health that have dangerous or deadly consequences (Paton, 2022). The extent to which social media influences health decisions remains a complex question, but you don't need to look far to see the impact that unregulated health information from social media is having on health (Zollo et al., 2024). Perhaps the most well-known and infamous example is the incorrect and disproven link between autism and MMR vaccines (Editors of The Lancet, 2010). The rise of anti-vaxxer influencers and vaccine hesitancy health information online, which find many of their origins in Wakefield's retracted and defunct paper, has had a direct consequence on global immunity to key diseases such as measles (Hussain et al., 2018).

It can be easy for healthcare professionals to dismiss people who use 'TikTok Health' to make decisions, such as vaccine-hesitant or anti-vaxxer patients, as a small ignorant group that can be ignored, but this too would be dangerous. First, such an assumption would be a big judgement that healthcare professionals are not really entitled to make. Why? Because healthcare professionals themselves are not immune to odd health beliefs. Vaccine hesitancy is particularly prominent in the field of nursing

(Wilson et al., 2020). Second, as ever with health, accurate health information and good clinical practice are only a small part of the overall health picture. Look no further than the United States, where the health secretary of Trump's 2024 cabinet, Robert F. Kennedy Jr, holds several health beliefs developed from unverified internet conspiracy theories (BBC Verify, 2024). Someone like this cannot be dismissed as an irrelevant loon, as he makes important decisions about health and healthcare for over 300 million people. The consequences of any healthcare policy that discredits the role of vaccines, to choose a real example from the Trump administration, could destroy decades of immunity to deadly disease globally. Heavy stuff.

Conclusion

Health beliefs are just that: beliefs. They are information that someone holds to be true, no matter how false or bizarre they may be. For the most part, people tend not to stray too far from accepted medical knowledge. Health beliefs can shape reasoning around decisions whether to see a doctor or how to engage with a suggested lifestyle change, but in general, when presented with a diagnosis and treatment plan, people will engage with it. Where we must tread carefully is in understanding that health beliefs are not just medical knowledge, but an important combination of personal, societal and clinical knowledge, which is brought together in a unique way for every single person when they shape their decisions about health. Societal beliefs around the validity of a health condition, or professional expectations that a condition should present in a particular way, can be damaging when adhered to in an overly strict way. Stigma around illness can result in shame, stopping patients from seeking help and completely changing their life forever.

Whether these beliefs are medically or even factually accurate is largely irrelevant. As difficult as it can be sometimes, as healthcare professionals, you must engage with even the most absurd of beliefs your patients may hold. For them, they are real beliefs, and they shape the decisions your patients make about their health. Denying or dismissing them out of hand, without at least trying to understand why the patient holds that belief, will likely mean that you lose their trust. If you are no longer a trusted source of health information, this can lead to poorer health and health outcomes for your patient down the road. Listening and politely engaging with their beliefs shows your patient that you view them as a person. You do not have to agree, and you may not get them to see your side, but you will have built trust, and you may find yourself rewarded in time with some changed beliefs and improved health.

Test Yourself

1. Define 'lay epidemiology'.
2. Doreen has had a cough for two weeks and is wondering whether she should see her doctor about it. She speaks to her husband, sister and co-worker, who all had the same cold, and asks them how long they were ill. They all tell her it took three weeks to get better, and so Doreen decides not to see her doctor about her cough. In doing so, what behaviour has Doreen displayed in order to make a decision about her health?

3. When Doreen finally does go to see her doctor, it turns out she has undiagnosed asthma. She is shocked. She has always been a bit 'chesty' but nothing that bothered her. She doesn't like her inhaler and only uses it when she thinks her asthma is really bad. What category of health belief does Doreen's behaviour fall into?
4. Identify and describe two limitations of Parsons' 'Sick Role' concept.
5. Biographical disruption identifies three ways that the onset of illness changes how we understand ourselves. What are these three ways?

References

Adams, S., Pill, R. and Jones, A. (1997). 'Medication, chronic illness and identity: The perspective of people with asthma.' *Social Science and Medicine* 45(2): 189–201. https://doi.org/10.1016/s0277-9536(96)00333-4

Barker, I., Steventon, A., Williamson, R. and Deeny, S.R. (2018). 'Self-management capability in patients with long-term conditions is associated with reduced healthcare utilisation across a whole health economy: Cross-sectional analysis of electronic health records.' *BMJ Quality & Safety* 27(12): 989–999. https://doi.org/10.1136/bmjqs-2017-007635

BBC Verify (2024). 'Fact-checking RFK Jr's views on health policy.' *BBC News*, 15th November. Available at: https://www.bbc.co.uk/news/articles/c0mzk2y41zvo

Bodryzlova, Y. and Moullec, G. (2023). 'Definitions of positive health: A systematic scoping review.' *Global Health Promotion* 30(3): 6–14. https://doi.org/10.1177/17579759221139802

Bury, M. (1982). 'Chronic illness as biographical disruption.' *Sociology of Health & Illness* 4: 167–182. https://doi.org/10.1111/1467-9566.ep11339939

Bury, M. and Monaghan, L. (2013). 'Illness narratives.' In *Illness narratives* [2nd Edition], edited by J. Gabe and L. Monaghan (pp. 82–86). SAGE Publications Ltd. https://doi.org/10.4135/9781526401687.n18

Charmaz, K. (1983). 'Loss of self: A fundamental form of suffering in the chronically ill.' *Sociology of Health & Illness* 5(2): 168–195. https://doi.org/10.1111/1467-9566.ep10491512

Corrigan, P.W., Larson, J.E. and Kuwabara, S.A. (2010). 'Social psychology of the stigma of mental illness: Public and self-stigma models.' In *Social psychological foundations of clinical psychology*, edited by J.E. Maddux and J.P. Tangney (pp. 51–68). The Guilford Press.

Doll, C.M., Michel, C., Betz, L.T., Schimmelmann, B.G. and Schultze-Lutter, F. (2022). 'The important role of stereotypes in the relation between mental health literacy and stigmatization of depression and psychosis in the community.' *Community Mental Health Journal* 58: 474–486. https://doi.org/10.1007/s10597-021-00842-5

Dunn, P., Ewbank, L. and Alderwick, H. (2023). 'Nine major challenges facing health and care in England.' *The Health Foundation*. Available at: https://www.health.org.uk/publications/long-reads/nine-major-challenges-facing-health-and-care-in-england

Editors of the Lancet (2010). 'Retraction—Ileal-lymphoid-nodular hyperplasia, non-specific colitis, and pervasive developmental disorder in children.' *The Lancet* 375(9713): 445. Available at: https://www.thelancet.com/journals/lancet/article/PIIS0140–6736(10)60175–4/abstract

Elliott, A.M., McAteer, A. and Hannaford, P.C. (2011). 'Revisiting the symptom iceberg in today's primary care: Results from a UK population survey.' *BMC Family Practice* 12: 16. https://doi.org/10.1186/1471-2296-12-16

Faircloth, C.A., Boylstein, C., Rittman, M., Young, M.E. and Gubrium, J. (2004). 'Sudden illness and biographical flow in narratives of stroke recovery.' *Sociology of Health & Illness* 26(2): 242–261. https://doi.org/10.1111/j.1467-9566.2004.00388.x

Godoy, M. (2023). 'Your kids are adorable germ vectors. Here's how often they get your household sick.' *NPR*, 26th January. Available at: https://www.npr.org/sections/health-shots/2023/01/26/1151333478/your-kids-are-adorable-germ-vectors-heres-how-often-they-get-your-household-sick [accessed 22nd August 2024].

Goffman, E. (1963). *Stigma notes on the management of spoiled identity*. Englewood Cliffs, NJ: Prentice-Hall Inc.

Gray, A. (2002). 'Stigma in psychiatry.' *Journal of the Royal Society of Medicine* 95: 72–76. https://doi.org/10.1177/014107680209500205

Hatzenbuehler, M.L. and Link, B.G. (2014). 'Introduction to the special issue on structural stigma and health.' *Social Science & Medicine* 103: 1–6. https://doi.org/10.1016/j.socscimed.2013.12.017

Hermetet, K. (n.d.). 'Dispelling myths about Tourette syndrome.' *Tourette Association of America*. Available at: https://tourette.org/debunking-myths-misconceptions/

Hussain, A., Ali, S., Ahmed, M. and Hussain, S. (2018). 'The anti-vaccination movement: A regression in modern medicine.' *Cureus* 10(7): e2919. https://doi.org/10.7759/cureus.2919

Ireland, L. (n.d.). 'Patient Trendscoping Study: What you need to know about patients of the future.' *Hall & Partners*. Available at: https://hallandpartners.com/perspectives/new-study-what-you-need-to-know-about-patients-of-the-future

Jafar, Z., Quick, J.D., Larson, H.J., Venegas-Vera, V., Napoli, P., Musuka, G., Dzinamarira, T., Meena, K.S., Kanmani, T.R. and Rimányi, E. (2023). 'Social media for public health: Reaping the benefits, mitigating the harms.' *Health Promotion Perspectives* 13(2): 105–112. https://doi.org/10.34172/hpp.2023.13

Kirkpatrick, S., Locock, L., Farre, A., Ryan, S., Salisbury, H. and McDonagh, J.E. (2018). 'Untimely illness: When diagnosis does not match age-related expectations.' *Health Expectations* 21(4): 730–740. https://doi.org/10.1111/hex.12669

Knaak, S., Mantler, E. and Szeto, A. (2017). 'Mental illness-related stigma in healthcare: Barriers to access and care and evidence-based solutions.' *Healthcare Management Forum* 30(2): 111–116. https://doi.org/10.1177/0840470416679413

Krahn, G.L., Robinson, A., Murray, A.J., Havercamp, S.M., Andridge, R., Arnold, L.E., Barnhill, J., Bodle, S., Boerner, E., Bonardi, A., Bourne, M.L., Brown, C., Buck, A., Burkett, S., Chapman, R., Cobranchi, C., Cole, C., Davies, D., Dresbach, T., Farr, J., Fay, M.L., Fletcher, R., Gertz, B., Hollway, J., Izzo, M., Lawrence-Slater, R., Lecavalier, L., Page, K., Perry, S., Poling, A., Rabidoux, P., Rice, R., Rosencrans, M., Ryan, M., Sanford, C., Schaeffer, C., Seeley, J., Shogren, K., Stepp, K., Straughter, M., Sucheston-Campbell, L., Tassé, M.J., Taylor, C., Walton, K., Wehmeyer, M., Williams, C. and Witwer, A. (2021). 'It's time to reconsider how we define health: Perspective from disability and chronic condition.' *Disability and Health Journal* 14(4). https://doi.org/10.1016/j.dhjo.2021.101129

Leonardi, M., Lee, H., Kostanjsek, N., Fornari, A., Raggi, A., Martinuzzi, A., Yáñez, M., Almborg, A.H., Fresk, M., Besstrashnova, Y., Shoshmin, A., Castro, S.S., Cordeiro, E.S., Cuenot, M., Haas, C., Maart, S., Maribo, T., Miller, J., Mukaino, M., Snyman, S., Trinks, U., Anttila, H., Paltamaa, J., Saleeby, P., Frattura, L., Madden, R., Sykes, C., Gool, C.H.V., Hrkal, J., Zvolský, M., Sládková, P., Vikdal, M., Harðardóttir, G.A., Foubert, J., Jakob, R., Coenen, M. and Kraus de Camargo, O. (2022). '20 Years of ICF-international classification of functioning, disability and health: Uses and applications around the world.' *International Journal of Environmental Research and Public Health* 19(18): 11321. https://doi.org/10.3390/ijerph191811321

Liddy, C., Blazkho, V. and Mill, K. (2014). 'Challenges of self-management when living with multiple chronic conditions: Systematic review of the qualitative literature.' *Canadian Family Physician* 60(12): 1123–1133. Available at: https://pmc.ncbi.nlm.nih.gov/articles/PMC4264810/

Macfarlane, H., Paton, A. and Bush, J. (2025). 'A qualitative exploration of the interaction between mental illness stigma and preparedness for practice in pharmacy students.' *Currents in Pharmacy Teaching and Learning* 17(3): 102271. https://doi.org/10.1016/j.cptl.2024.102271

McQuater, K. (2023). 'Report shows influence of social media for healthcare information.' *Research Live*, 15th February. Available at: https://www.research-live.com/article/news/report-shows-influence-of-social-media-for-healthcare-information/id/5109082

Mental Health Foundation (2021). *Stigma and discrimination*. Available at: https://www.mentalhealth.org.uk/explore-mental-health/a-z-topics/stigma-and-discrimination

Mind (2020). *Mental health facts and statistics*. Available at: https://www.mind.org.uk/information-support/types-of-mental-health-problems/mental-health-facts-and-statistics/

Mind (n.d.). *Facts and figures about racism and mental health*. Available at: https://www.mind.org.uk/about-us/our-strategy/becoming-a-truly-anti-racist-organisation/facts-and-figures-about-racism-and-mental-health/

Nuffield Trust (2025). *Care and support for long term conditions*. Available at: https://www.nuffieldtrust.org.uk/resource/care-and-support-for-long-term-conditions

Nutbeam, D. (1998). 'Health promotion glossary.' *Health Promotion International* 13(4): 349–364. https://doi.org/10.1093/heapro/13.4.349

Office for National Statistics (n.d.). *Population estimates*. Available at: https://www.ons.gov.uk/peoplepopulationandcommunity/populationandmigration/populationestimates

Parsons, T. (1951). 'Illness and the role of the physician: A sociological perspective.' *American Journal of Orthopsychiatry* 21(3): 452–460. https://doi.org/10.1111/j.1939-0025.1951.tb00003.x

Paton, A. (2022). 'The surveillance of pregnant bodies in the age of digital health: Ethical dilemmas.' In *The Routledge handbook on feminist bioethics*, edited by W.A. Rogers, J. Leach Scully, S.M. Carter, V.A. Entwistle and C. Mills. New York: Routledge.

Paton, A., Armstrong, N., Smith, L. and Lotto, R. (2020). 'Parents' decision-making following diagnosis of a severe congenital anomaly in pregnancy: Practical, theoretical and ethical tensions.' *Social Science and Medicine* 266: 113362. https://doi.org/10.1016/j.socscimed.2020.113362

Rudd, R.E. (2015). 'The evolving concept of health literacy: New directions for health literacy studies.' *Journal of Communication in Healthcare* 8(1): 7–9. https://doi.org/10.1179/1753806815Z.000000000105

Sartorius, N. (2006). 'The meanings of health and its promotion.' *Croatian Medical Journal* 47(4): 662–664. Available at: https://pmc.ncbi.nlm.nih.gov/articles/PMC2080455/

Sensky, T. (1996). 'Eliciting lay beliefs across cultures: Principles and methodology.' *British Journal of Cancer* 74(XXIX): S63–S65. Available at: https://pmc.ncbi.nlm.nih.gov/articles/PMC2149866/

Stuart, H. (2006). 'Media portrayal of mental illness and its treatments: What effect does it have on people with mental illness?' *CNS Drugs* 20(2): 99–106. https://doi.org/10.2165/00023210-200620020-00002

Sykes, C.R., Maribo, T., Stallinga, H.A. and Heerkens, Y. (2021). 'Remodeling of the ICF: A commentary.' *Disability and Health Journal* 14(1): 100978. https://doi.org/10.1016/j.dhjo.2020.100978

Tatchell, P. (2017). 'Don't fall for the myth that it's 50 years since we decriminalised homosexuality.' *The Guardian*, 23rd May. Available at: https://www.theguardian.com/commentisfree/2017/may/23/fifty-years-gay-liberation-uk-barely-four-1967-act

Wahl, O.F. (1995). *Media madness: Public images of mental illness*. Piscataway, NJ: Rutgers University Press.

Wilson, R., Zaytseva, A., Bocquier, A., Nokri, A., Fressard, L., Chamboredon, P., Carbonaro, C., Bernardi, S., Dubé, E. and Verger, P. (2020). 'Vaccine hesitancy and self-vaccination behaviors among nurses in southeastern France.' *Vaccine* 38(5): 1144–1151. https://doi.org/10.1016/j.vaccine.2019.11.018

World Health Organisation (2001). *International classification of functioning, disability and health (ICF)*. Available at: https://iris.who.int/bitstream/handle/10665/42407/9241545429-eng.pdf [accessed 20th August 2024].

World Health Organisation (2018). *International classification of functioning, disability and health (ICF)*. Available at: https://www.who.int/standards/classifications/international-classification-of-functioning-disability-and-health

World Health Organisation (n.d.). *Health literacy*. Available at: https://www.who.int/teams/health-promotion/enhanced-wellbeing/ninth-global-conference/health-literacy

Zollo, F., Baronchelli, A., Betsch, C., Delmastro, M. and Quattrociocchi, W. (2024). 'Understanding the complex links between social media and health behaviour.' *British Medical Journal* 385: e075645. https://doi.org/10.1136/bmj-2023-075645

Health-related behaviours

It should be obvious by now that while medicine and health have important clinical components, at the end of the day you are working with humans, not machines. As such, they will ultimately only do what they want to do. Their behaviours around health are subject to their circumstances and their beliefs, and this will influence the way they act with regards to their health. It can be helpful to understand the existing theories of health behaviour when supporting your patients: these can either help you understand why patients act as they do, or provide patients with tools to change their behaviour in ways that will better facilitate a healthy life for themselves. In this chapter, I will review the more prominent and pertinent theories of health-related behaviour for your practice. I will also explain why the relationship you have with your patients influences these behaviours.

Health-related behaviours

The theories of health-related behaviour cover three things:

1. How we can predict people's behaviour with regards to health.
2. How we can change people's behaviour with regards to health.
3. How we can manage people's behaviour with regards to health.

These three goals aim to prevent disease, return people to health and promote health. Health-related behaviour is so important that understanding how to manage it can be considered a key competency when it comes to healthcare, and guidance and guidelines on demonstrating and employing them come up again and again in the GMC, NMC, GPhC and in National Institute for Health and Care Excellence (NICE) guidance (NICE, 2014).

So what are health-related behaviours? Essentially, a health-related behaviour is any behaviour that has a consequence for health and/or illness. We often think of

DOI: 10.4324/9781032677552-4

health-related behaviours as being behaviours that either promote health, known as positive/health-promoting behaviours, or behaviours that lead to poor health and/or illness, known as negative/health-risk behaviours. For example, smoking is a classic negative/health-risk behaviour, while regular exercise is a classic positive/health-promoting behaviour. Other seemingly clinical activities also constitute health-related behaviours. For example, getting an STI test or keeping up to date with vaccinations are positive health-related behaviours. As a general rule, in medicine we want people to engage in positive/health-promoting behaviours and limit or avoid negative/health-risk behaviours.

You might be wondering why we should care about health-related behaviours. After all, there has so far been a strong 'you do you' message in this book when it comes to patient choice. While it is very much the case that patients will make their own decisions that impact their health one way or another, it cannot be denied that this comes with consequences. Globally, health-related behaviours are the highest contributors to overall disease burden (Woolf and Aron, 2013). If we take a well-recognised negative health-related behaviour, tobacco smoking, we can see the extent to which the way people act when it comes to health can have significant consequences. Smoking is responsible for 71% of all lung cancer death and close to half (41%) of all chronic respiratory disease—and it is not just our lungs that suffer when we smoke, as smoking is also responsible for 10% of ischaemic heart disease deaths (World Health Organisation, n.d.). The United Kingdom has a particular issue with this; about a quarter of all deaths would have been avoidable had patients engaged in lifestyle changes (Office for National Statistics, 2024; Meikle, 2015), and this number has remained steady for almost ten years.

Psychological theories of health behaviours

Over the years, the field of psychology has developed theories to help us better understand why people do what they do. It is important to remember that these are just theories, and people do not always fit neatly into theories, but understanding these psychological concepts can be helpful in clinical practice, as this knowledge can be used to support patients to change their health behaviours.

There are several theories that can and do fill textbooks, but for our purposes we will focus on six theories most relevant to healthcare. These are sometimes also called 'models' of health behaviour. Again, no theory or model can *make* someone change how they act. Instead, think of these theories as tools to support behaviour change, as they provide ways and techniques to predict behaviour in certain circumstances and influence health-promoting behaviour. In both instances, the theories can support change at the individual or population level. Finally, as in most areas where multiple theories exist, there is no discipline-wide agreement on which is the most effective. Instead of thinking about them in a prescriptive way, that is this problem equals this theory, instead think of them as potential tools in a toolbox and consider which might be the most effective for each person. It will of course be different for different people most of the time.

Classical conditioning

Perhaps, without realising it, you already know the basics of classical conditioning because you have likely heard of its most famous example: the Pavlovian Response.

Pavlov was a Russian scientist who tried to understand human reflexes and spent most of his life interested in our digestion. He worked a lot with dogs, and in doing so made a significant discovery. He discovered that the ringing of a bell, carried out while giving the dogs their food, created an association for the dogs between the bell and their saliva glands—meaning they would start to salivate at the sound of the bell, even when there was no food. Leaving aside Pavlov's questionable animal rights beliefs and strange propensity to be judgemental about his dog subjects (his notes label some of them as 'lazy', 'greedy', etc.), Pavlov spent his life studying our reflexes and helped us to understand the associations we create with the world around us (McCabe, 2014).

The association of the dog with the bell is an example of classic conditioning, where a new behaviour is learnt through the process of association (Thrailkill and Rey, 2024). By linking two stimuli together, in this case the bell and the food, a new learned response is created through classical conditioning. This discovery by Pavlov showed that unconditional responses (e.g. salivating is a natural response to the presence of food) to unconditional stimuli (the food) could become conditioned responses to conditioned stimuli (e.g. the bell) (Thrailkill and Rey, 2024). In this way, classical conditioning subverts natural responses to new stimuli.

Of course, unless you are a vet who has grabbed the wrong book off the shelf, you may be thinking that what dogs do when they hear bells is not really helpful for clinical practice in humans. *Au contraire*. Humans share these unconditional responses and so we can also be subject to classical conditioning.

Let's talk about how this works. If someone is a prolific snacker and they are looking to cut down on snacking, they can try only eating in one place in their house—their kitchen table, for example. If they're indulging their snack cravings all over the house, they are creating associations with eating in multiple locations. Over time, this causes a conditioned response with multiple triggers. If they only eat in one spot, like the kitchen table, then, over time, only that location will elicit the conditioned response of the desire to eat. If they avoid the table, they'll probably snack less.

For the most part we have unconscious associations with things—meaning we don't intend to associate one thing with another, but, over time, the repetitive grouping together of cues with responses creates the association for us. This becomes a problem when these associations trigger negative/health-risk behaviours.

Classical conditioning can help us to understand why we associate cues with behaviours, and so most of the work in classical conditioning to promote behaviour change is centred around breaking the habits that cause the unconscious response, avoiding the associated cues or changing the association entirely. The snacking example shows how classic conditioning can help with lifestyle changes by facilitating the learning of new behaviours. While I have chosen a low-stakes example, it is easy to see how this approach might support someone trying to cut down on harmful behaviours such as drug or alcohol consumption. The most extreme form of behaviour change that classical conditioning provides is that of aversion therapy. Buckle up because this is a truly extreme approach that has not always been used for 'good', so indulge me in a brief foray into medicine's murky history with classical conditioning.

Aversion therapy
The basic concept of aversion therapy is rather simple: use negative stimulus to stop bad behaviour. It takes what we know about conditioning behaviour from Pavlov and his

peers and uses the same concept, but in a negative way, to dissuade people from engaging in certain health behaviours deemed undesirable or risky (APA, 2018). These days, aversion therapy is employed when appropriate to help with addictions such as alcoholism (CMS, n.d.). By pairing together alcohol with medication that induces unpleasant stimuli (often vomiting or severe nausea), the person eventually associates alcohol with the unpleasant stimuli and stops drinking alcohol altogether in order to avoid feeling that way in the future. It is the exact same concept as Pavlov and his dogs with their bell, except that the association is negative. There is no denying that aversion therapy is an unpleasant way to alter behaviour, but it does appear to provide results. However, for many it does nothing to alter the circumstances that have brought about the behaviours, and thus half the problem remains unsolved.

Additionally, who decides what health behaviours are undesirable? Some may seem blindingly obvious: smoking and alcohol dependency do known, long-lasting damage to our bodies. However, as we discussed in earlier chapters, not all behaviour is truly risky, and aversion therapy is a cautionary tale of why those in medicine must always question why something is deemed to be harmful.

Let me explain. Throughout the 1960s and 1970s, the aversion therapy heyday if you will, it was predominantly used to 'treat' homosexuality, which was considered by medicine and much of the American and European society as a deviant health behaviour that required correcting (Minton, 2002). This went beyond simple stigma or shame about being homosexual. The Diagnostic Statistical Manual of the American Psychological Association and the WHO's International Classification of Diseases both labelled homosexuality as a mental disorder (Minton, 2002). Aversion therapy was the treatment of choice for this 'mental illness', and the same principles used today when treating alcoholism with aversion therapy were deployed to 'cure' people of their risky health behaviours brought on by their attraction to the same gender.

Aversion therapy is a good example of why, when discussing how to support behavioural change in patients, it is important to pause and ask yourself: 'Why is this health behaviour considered undesirable?' What is driving the beliefs that the behaviour must be changed? Most of the time there are clear clinical reasons why, but what is considered health-promoting versus health-risky is not just decided by clinical parameters—societal norms and beliefs shape these definitions too and, as a result, shape clinical intervention.

Unfortunately, aversion therapy for homosexuality took decades to fall out of fashion and traumatised countless people who were simply trying to fit into a society that could not and would not let them live as their authentic selves. Aversion therapy for homosexuality is no longer an accepted or recognised medical practice, but it lives on as 'conversion therapy' offered worldwide by unscrupulous providers (Davison et al., 2024).

Operant conditioning

Developed by B.F. Skinner (1937), operant conditioning modifies behaviour through reinforcement in the form of punishment or reward. Like Pavlov, Skinner was working with animals and observed that animals learn behaviour based on the consequences of that behaviour. He theorised that these consequences could be used to modify the behaviour. Humans, being of course animals, are also subject to this relationship

(Skinner, 1963). Skinner argued that if a particular behaviour is reinforced through reward or the removal of punishment, people will engage more frequently and more willingly with that behaviour. If a particular behaviour is punished or a reward removed, people will engage less or be less willing to engage in that behaviour. The correct use of this system can modify behaviour (Skinner, 1963).

Anyone who has ever had a 'reward' chart as a child, or organised one for their own children, will know this system well.[1] We actually use this type of behavioural change approach all the time and often don't even think of it as a 'behavioural change' mechanism at all. Consider the last time you cut something out, such as takeaway coffee, for a few months in order to save up for a holiday or something you really wanted. This is a very mild but effective form of operant conditioning. More recently there have been several interesting uses of operant conditioning to help with smoking cessation, such as the free NHS app Quit Smoking. The Quit Smoking app tracks how much a user saves for every day of not smoking. In doing so it creates a reward (money saved) for the behaviour change (not smoking). The app tracks the progress and the overall amount of money saved, thus reinforcing a positive reward for modified behaviour (NHS, n.d.). The Quit Smoking app is not just a useful example of operant conditioning for health behaviour modification; it also shows how useful understanding health behaviours can be for public health and health promotion, promoting healthy behaviours at the individual and population levels.

Like classical conditioning, operant conditioning does not always address the full cause of the problematic behaviour, nor can it always deal with the scale of that behaviour. Both classical and operant conditioning view humans as basic creatures who can be trained, rewarded or punished into changes in their behaviour—but of course we are not. As we have seen in the first few chapters of this book, people make decisions based on a wide variety of information, the detail of which is specific to them and is also influenced by cultural, social, systemic and commercial determinants of health. We are also all different in the extent to which we are open to this type of learning. Neither approach considers the differences in cognitive processes that every person has and, in particular, the strong immediacy of the reward for many health-risk behaviours like junk food, alcohol and drugs.

Ultimately, neither classical nor operant conditioning can change living conditions or reduce the trauma that can trigger poor health behaviour. They do not make healthy food more rewarding. Only sometimes do they give us more money to make changes to our circumstances, providing the resources to change health-risk behaviours. Furthermore, for some people, rewards and punishments need to be of such a high magnitude to modify behaviour that it may be impossible to achieve behaviour change, as was seen when researchers tried to improve drug abstinence rates in Baltimore by incentivising the avoidance of drugs (Silverman, 2004). As I said at the beginning of this chapter, at the end of the day, people will still do what they want regardless of the consequences.

Social-cognition models of health behaviour

Social-cognition models of health behaviour are constructed around the idea that we learn by observing what other people do and then imitating and modelling that behaviour (Bandura, 1977). There is still an element of reward and punishment, in that we observe which behaviours are rewarded and look to imitate and model those, while avoiding behaviours that we observe as being punished (Bandura, 1977). Interestingly this observation can take place in person or through media. We are more likely to model behaviour when we trust the model of that behaviour, for example people with high status (leaders, celebrities, parents), or when we perceive them to be like us (peer groups). As a result, this can help us learn good or harmful health behaviours. If the behaviour is not observed as being punished and the model is important to us (for example, a parent who smokes with no negative consequences), then we may also learn to model and imitate harmful behaviours, for example the child will go on to smoke.

Cognitive dissonance theory
Cognitive dissonance is a mental discomfort that occurs when someone's behaviour is not consistent with their beliefs. A classic example is people who smoke even though they know smoking causes cancer, which results in feelings of shame or guilt. Leon Festinger argued that we can use cognitive dissonance to help improve behaviour because people do not like the discomfort of dissonance and will act to reduce it in some way (Festinger, 1957). Festinger studied a cult who believed the earth would be destroyed by a flood, focusing on what happened in the cult when the promised flood never came. He argued that humans want their beliefs, attitudes and behaviours to align and will avoid changes in these three aspects that cause them to become mis-aligned (dissonance). He called this the principle of cognitive consistency.

Humans want cognitive consistency, and when it comes to health behaviours, we can exploit this need to bring about changes in beliefs or behaviours to avoid dissonance. The best way to do this is through health promotion campaigns. A good example of this is the changes to cigarette packaging in the last 20 years to include those nightmare-inducing photos of black lungs and cancerous mouth tumours. These have been designed with cognitive dissonance in mind—the idea being that if someone knows they shouldn't smoke, but they still do, the images increase the discomfort and tension of their cognitive dissonance to the point that they may alter their behaviour to realign their beliefs and behaviours and return to a cognitive consistency.

Of course, the theory cannot predict that the behaviour will change—the beliefs could change instead, so as to accommodate the continuation of the behaviour. Festinger observed this amongst the most devoted members of the cult: when no flood appeared, they argued that the earth was not destroyed as foretold due to the faithfulness of the cult members. In less crazy terms: they changed their beliefs, rather than changing their behaviour by leaving the cult (Festinger, 1957). In this way, cognitive dissonance theory does not necessarily change beliefs or behaviours in a way that leads to more health-promoting behaviours; it can go the other way too.

The health belief model
The Health Belief Model was developed in the mid-twentieth century to help both explain and predict health behaviours in people. The model assumes that people will engage in health-related behaviours (Hochbaum et al., 1952) if they believe that:

1. They are susceptible to a condition/illness/disease (perceived susceptibility)
2. The condition will have serious consequences for them (perceived severity)

3. The behaviour will benefit them by reducing their susceptibility or the severity of the condition (perceived benefits)
4. These benefits will outweigh barriers to engaging in that behaviour (perceived barriers)
5. They can engage in the behaviour successfully to get the outcome they want (self-efficacy)

The factors that actually trigger a person to engage in the behaviour can be internal (for example the appearance of a symptom) or external (for example education or advice from a doctor). These factors are called Cues to Action (Wethington et al., 2015). Interestingly, the model recognises that the social determinants of health influence individual health beliefs and the resulting behaviours (sometimes referred to as Modifying Factors), making it a more holistic model (Wethington et al., 2015).

Theory of planned behaviour

Ajzen proposed that in order to know or predict whether people will engage in a particular behaviour, we need to know whether they in fact intend to do that behaviour (Ajzen, 1991). This intention is predicated on three key things (Ajzen, 1991):

1. The person's attitude towards the behaviour
2. The subjective norms around that behaviour
3. Perceived behavioural control

Let's look at these three aspects in more detail, taking the example of encouraging someone to eat more fruit and vegetables. First, you would want to know the person's attitude towards eating more fruit and vegetables. If the person has a positive attitude towards eating more fruit and vegetables and perhaps even enjoys eating them, this will positively influence their intention to eat more. The subjective norms of eating more fruit and vegetables are also important. By this, I mean the beliefs of the people around the person considering a change in behaviour—not only those immediately around them, like friends and family, but also the cultural norms with which they live. If those around the person also eat lots of fruit and vegetables and think it is a good thing, this is again more likely to have a positive influence on the person's intention to change their behaviour. Finally, perceived behavioural control—meaning the person's own belief that they will be able to engage in the desired behaviour effectively (sometimes called self-efficacy)—will positively influence intention. Using our example, this would be the person's confidence in their own ability to buy and eat more fruit and vegetables in a consistent manner.

However, it is not always as straightforward as this. We need only look at ourselves and remember all the times our own attitudes, subjective norms and perceived behavioural control have led to intentions to change behaviour, only for that behaviour to remain unchanged. This is known as the intention-behaviour gap (Faries, 2016). In recent years, in response to this gap, past behaviour has been added to the overall model of the Theory of Planned Behaviour as a way of improving the predictability that intention will lead to a person actually changing their behaviour (Hagger et al., 2016).

Of course, we know that past behaviour is influenced by the social world around us. Luckily the Theory of Planned Behaviour has moved with the conceptual times on this, widening out the sphere of influence on behaviour to include 'socio-structural varia-bles' as important sources of information that shape behaviour (Hagger and Hamilton, 2021). These variables are, of course, our good friends the social and structural deter-minants of health. In particular, Haggard and their team found that when education, income, age and gender were included in the model, it increased the accuracy of the overall model of predicting behaviour (Hagger and Hamilton, 2021).

Limitations of the social-cognition models

While all the models explained here can help modify behaviour, they make big assump-tions about humans that are simply not the reality for most people. They assume that all people consume, process and act on health information in the same way and that they have the same access to health information. We know from the previous chapters that this is not the case—far from it. The way that people access, consume and use health information varies wildly. The models also assume that people place a high priority on their health and will always want to act in its best interest. However, many people, for a wide variety of reasons, do not prioritise their health, so the incentives for engaging in positive health behaviours are low. There is also no discussion of the resources required to engage in the desired behaviour—financial, emotional or otherwise. Neither is emo-tion considered a factor, even though it plays a significant part in our day-to-day deci-sion-making. There are also practical limitations to these theories—notably that they can tell people that they should change behaviour and what behaviour to change, but offer no guidance or advice on *how* to change. This means that, at best, they can pre-dict an intention to change, but not necessarily that a particular behaviour will actually change.

Integrative models of behaviour

As a result of these limitations, attempts have been made to develop more integrated models that focus on individual behaviour change to improve health behaviours. These models consider broader factors in terms of influencing behaviour change. For exam-ple, different people tend to be at different stages of readiness for change. However, as with previous models in this chapter, the ability for integrative models to predict behav-iour is modest at best. There are so many variables that make up a person, meaning that it remains difficult to find a model that can adequately account for differences in behaviour type, context, population targeted, motivation, emotion—the list is as end-less and complex as humans. Of course, all of this can further vary with just a small change in circumstances (for example having a bit more money to spend on health behaviours such as healthier food) or more significant changes in context such as the COVID-19 pandemic.

The transtheoretical model

The Transtheoretical Model is one of the most well-known and used integrated mod-els, though it mostly goes by its more common name: the Stages of Change Model. Developed by Prochaska and DiClemente in 1983 to support smoking cessation, the basic concept of this model is that when people want to change their behaviour, they go through different stages to achieve the change (Prochaska and DiClemente, 1983). At each stage, a person needs different resources to support them in developing the

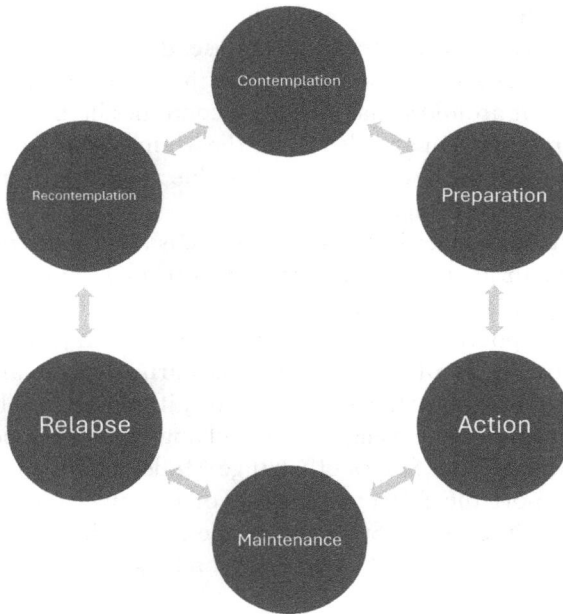

Figure 4.1 The Stages of Change Model.

behaviours needed for that particular stage, which should enable them to move forward to the next stage of change. The model promotes decisional balance and the confidence to make better choices, avoid temptation and make healthier decisions.

The Stages of Change Model has six stages. In theory, they follow one after another; however, the overall model is a cycle of behaviour, not linear. Figure 4.1 shows how the stages interact with each other.

In some cases, people spend longer in one stage, or may skip stages altogether (Prochaska and Di Clemente, 1983). A person can also move forward or backward between the stages. So how does it work to change behaviour? Let's consider the model with regards to social media use and mental health.

In the Precontemplation Stage, the person may simply be aware that they do not feel mentally well. Something is not right. Perhaps they have higher levels of anxiety or feel down. Behaviour change is not on their mind at this stage.

The Contemplation Stage sees a recognition that this feeling of unwellness may be linked to the person's social media use, and they contemplate, that is start to think, that maybe there needs to be a change in their social media use in the future to improve their mental wellbeing.

In the Preparation Stage, no action is taken. Instead, the focus is on planning the future strategy. A decision has been taken to do something and this stage helps identify what that something is. It may involve getting friends to agree to use social media less, or activities such as searching and reading about the impact of social media use on mental wellbeing. It normally involves identifying future actions, such as researching and choosing an app to limit social media use.

Once the person starts engaging with the actions they have identified in the Preparation Stage above—limiting social media use, deleting social media apps, using apps to create boundaries around use—they enter the Action Stage of the model.

As the new behaviour around social media use continues in the long term, it becomes the 'new normal' for the person and they enter the Maintenance Stage. The idea of the Maintenance Stage is that the new behaviour is stable and the person can maintain the changes they have made over time.

However, as with all changes in behaviour, there is always the risk of returning to the unhealthy behaviour at some point—known as relapse. This is why the Stages of Change Model is a cycle, as a person can relapse at any given time. When this happens, they always have the opportunity to return to the Precontemplation Stage and begin the journey anew. Equally, as all stages do not necessarily apply to all people, they may simply jump back to the Action Stage—for example, if they relapse but want to implement the same actions they were using before to change their behaviour.

As an integrated model, the Stages of Change Model allows the other models discussed earlier to support the different stages. For example, the Theory of Planned Behaviour can support the Action Stage, while the Health Behaviour Model is useful for supporting the Maintenance and Contemplation Stages. This is a hallmark of integrated models.

Strengths and limitations of the transtheoretical model
The strength of this model is that it recognises that everyone is different, with different circumstances. As a result, while many people may want to adopt better health behaviours, they will be at different stages of readiness for doing so. The model promotes recognition of these differences and seeks to tailor its interventions to the particular stage in which the person finds themself. It also recognises the limitations of all models in promoting lasting change. In allowing for the relapse stage of the cycle, the Stages of Change Model is a more realistic account of what achieving behavioural change really looks like. In this way, it normalises the important fact that when learning a new behaviour, mistakes will be made. That is how we learn!

PRIME theory
PRIME theory is a relatively new theory in the health behaviour field. Similarly to behavioural learning theories, this theory suggests that people have external and internal stimuli that cause behaviours or behavioural change (West, 2007). However, it is not a direct cause (stimulus) and effect (behavioural change) relationship. Instead, PRIME theory argues that the stimulus causes people to go through various steps that ultimately lead to a response, which is the behaviour change (West, 2007). The letters in PRIME stand for the following steps (West, 2007):

Plans: The intentions of the person
Response: The behaviour or action of the person
Impulses: The urges the person has to act one way or another
Motives: The wants or desires of the person, which may not be the healthiest choice
Evaluation: The person's own health beliefs

Frustratingly, the order of PRIME is not the order in which West suggests the stages happen. Instead, the process is similar to the Stages of Change Model. It looks a little like this:

The stimulus sets off Plans ⇄ Evaluation ⇄ Motives ⇄ Impulses ⇄ Response

At any point the person can slip backwards, often as a result of stimuli, so again, this model is not as linear as it may appear (West and Brown, 2013).

There are four main assumptions in the PRIME theory (West and Brown, 2013):

First, it is necessary to understand people's moment-to-moment behaviour—how they effectively decide what they are doing from one moment to the next. Without this understanding, it is impossible to understand long-term influences on behaviour. To go back to our social media use example, it is necessary to understand the 'small' daily decisions people make, such as why they choose to scroll social media instead of doing something else, in order to understand how to improve use in the future.

The second assumption is a biggie: that thanks to our brain's plasticity, we are all capable of learning and changing our behaviour as a result of that learning. Again, when it comes to social media use, the assumption that PRIME makes here is that people can learn to interact with social media in different ways then they have done before.

The third key assumption of PRIME theory is who we understand ourselves to be: our self-identity. Our self-identity plays a big part in our motives and plans and thus significantly impacts on our responses to stimuli. This is because our self-identification drives our beliefs, and as we learnt earlier, people don't like their behaviour and their beliefs to be at odds—this is called cognitive dissonance.

Self-identity is a good assumption for us to consider alongside the social media example. For many people, who they are and what they believe is strongly tied to their social media use. They may take significant self-worth from their interactions on social media or actively shape their identity around the way they present themselves on social media. Their beliefs about that relationship, and its ability to change, are critical for this third assumption that PRIME makes.

Finally, PRIME assumes that people's motivational systems are relatively simple processes—that they are ultimately focused on the balance between a desire or urge and the decision to make a different, ideally healthier, choice. Again, when translated into our social media use example, this is about balancing the urge to use social media versus the knowledge that healthier social media habits are likely better for one's wellbeing.

PRIME tries to integrate more concepts into our understanding of behaviour than many previous theories. It also looks to bring together emotions, motivation, context, self-identity, etc. with existing concepts of behaviour. This is a very recent model, so at present its efficacy to predict and change behaviour remains largely unknown.

COM-B model of behaviour

The COM-B model, developed by Michie et al. (2011), focuses on three main requirements for behaviour change (Michie et al., 2011):

First, people must have the capability (C), meaning the physical and psychological skill or ability, to perform the behaviour. This normally means that people have the knowledge and physical ability to some extent.

Second, they must have the opportunity (O), meaning the physical and social resources, including time, to perform the behaviour.

Both capability and opportunity drive people's motivation (M) to perform the behaviour. This includes both automative motivation, meaning impulses, and reflective motivation, for example a plan or desire to perform the behaviour. There can be influences between and across these three elements, but at its heart, COM-B seeks to simplify our understanding of behaviour.

In short, a person needs capability, opportunity and motivation to perform behaviours (B)—hence COM-B, which stands for each element. Thus, if you want to change people's behaviour, you must promote and support change in people's capability, opportunity and motivation. The COM-B model can be used with the Behaviour Change Wheel, which helps identify appropriate interventions for tackling a lack of capacity, opportunity or motivation (Michie et al., 2011). These can also be used to influence health policy and practice.

Behaviour change and the COVID-19 pandemic

Behavioural models are not only useful for supporting individual changes in behaviour; they can also have wider uses. This was the case during the COVID-19 pandemic. The Scientific Advisory Group for Emergencies in England (SAGE) has a specific behavioural science sub-group, SPI-B (Scientific Pandemic Insights Group on Behaviours), that provides advice to the UK government; it had a direct influence on policy and guidance during the pandemic (UK Parliament, 2020; Michie et al., 2021).

This group provided useful insights on the implementation of the key infection control measures which we are all so familiar with now. Namely:

- School closures
- Home isolation of symptomatic people
- Voluntary household quarantine
- Social distancing

While aspects of each key measure were (and still remain) disputed, behavioural science and its models were a key component of the decisions made during the first two years of the pandemic.

As part of their work, SPI-B were commissioned by the Cabinet Office of the UK Government to identify the appropriate behaviour model to promote infection control behaviours in the population that would limit COVID-19 transmission in the long term (Michie et al., 2021).

COM-B and its associated Behavioural Change Wheel were identified as the best models to adopt. Examples of the kinds of strategies recommended under the COM-B model included (Michie et al., 2021):

- Capability: Multichannel information and communication campaigns, in a wide variety of places such as schools and workplaces, that explain the importance of ventilation and face coverings (for example) to reduce transmission

---

- Opportunity: Ensuring sufficient financial support and resources for people to be able to comply with behaviour changes, such as self-isolation periods
- Motivation: Using a variety of techniques such as targeted training and resources, even TV advertising, to build habits and routines linked to behaviours that reduce transmission, such as always bringing a face mask when leaving the house

Nudge theory

Nudge theory should be a familiar concept to you, even if you don't necessarily know what it is. If you've ever ordered food at McDonald's, you will have been subjected to a nudge that is pretty commonplace in the food industry: asking if you would like to upgrade your order to a larger size. If you're as old as me, you might even remember the famous 'Supersize' tagline. Nudge theory assumes that about 80% of all human behaviour is automatic, and that we can tap into this automation to change behaviour. By this, Thaler and Sustein (2008), who developed the concept, mean that people unconsciously respond to cues in their environment that shape their choices without ever realising it—what they call choice architecture.

To 'nudge' someone towards a different behaviour, it is necessary to make simple changes to the choice architecture that people encounter. A good example of this is the 'Now Wash Your Hands' signs that we frequently see in public toilets across the United Kingdom. The idea is that placing this sign somewhere that everyone sees, such as above the sink or on the back of a toilet stall door, will prompt people to make the decision to wash their hands without thinking about it.

(By the way, should you, for some reason, require more motivation than simple hygiene to wash your hands, remember that most public toilets contain on average 500,000 bacterial cells per square inch on bathroom surfaces within one hour of use (Gibbons et al., 2015). So, really, wash your hands!)

Nudges have to be appropriately tailored to both the environment and the desired behaviour, and so they must possess two qualities to be successful. First, it has to be easy to make the desired choice, and second, it should improve people's motivation to make that choice. Returning again to social media use, a good example of a nudge are the apps that require us to act in some way to access social media—for example using a time monitor to track how much time someone spends on social media or a 'pause' reminder after the app has been open for a certain amount of time. All of these create a new choice architecture within which people make different choices about the way they use social media.

Nudge theory is popular across several disciplines, not just healthcare, and there is some justification for this popularity. In health, at least, a meta-analysis has shown that nudge theory could be the key to a healthier public, as it can improve diet choices (Arno and Thomas, 2016). The potential for nudges to improve overall population health is thus a real possibility.

Everything tastes better than being thin

The thing is, despite all the potential of the models described in this chapter, we still don't take as much action to improve our health as we should. Why is that? Well, the

COM-B model is probably best for helping us understand why people don't do things: they may lack the capability. For example, a person may not know that social media use can have a negative impact on their mental wellbeing. People may also lack the opportunity to change their behaviour. Again, focusing on social media, it may be that social media use is somehow integral to a person's job or wider social life, so they don't necessarily have the option to step back from it. Alternatively, there may be a lack of motivation to change the way they use social media because they find enjoyment in using it.

An unfortunate fact of life is that a lot of the tasty, fun, enjoyable behaviours that provide immediate hits of happiness can also be unhealthy if performed in the wrong way. Health behaviours are often perceived as (or just are, let's be honest) boring, difficult and, if running is as awful for you as it is for me, downright unpleasant.

(NB: Should you ever see me on a nature path looking like I'm in the throes of a heart attack—never fear. I'm just training for a fun run someone has roped me into.)

Who is really in charge of our health? Understanding the power dynamics in the healthcare professional-patient relationship

All this talk of models of health behaviour and trying to get people to change their ways may have you wondering who is really in charge when it comes to health behaviour. That's a tricky question to answer. Just as the social world impacts on beliefs and behaviours, the way people understand their health, construct beliefs about it and then act according to those beliefs must be understood within the context of the healthcare professional-patient relationship. This relationship is not neutral and is as important for influencing behaviour as the psychological models that describe health behaviour. It contains several layers of power that influence both the people in the relationship (Paton, 2017). Like all relationships, it is governed by transactions and the currency of transactions. In the case of medicine, the currency is information and understanding (Paton, 2017). This sets up an inevitable power dynamic in the clinical encounter, whereby the healthcare professional is assumed to have more power because, again, it is assumed they have a greater understanding of clinical knowledge (Paton, 2017). For a better understanding of the influence of the healthcare professional-patient relationship in the clinical encounter, and by extension the impact this relationship has on health beliefs and behaviours, let us briefly look at the different ways of understanding that relationship.

Broadly speaking, there are four 'types' of possible healthcare professional-patient relationship (Morgan, 2008). Of course (and you knew there was going to be an 'of course'), these are artificial categories that can help to understand the dynamics of a relationship, but they do not necessarily reflect all possible healthcare professional-patient relationships. In fact, a single relationship, even one single clinical encounter, can contain all four 'types' and more.

Paternalism

Paternalism is perhaps the most well-known, but also vilified, of the relationship types. In this model, the physician is chiefly in control and makes decisions without input from the patient. It is unsurprising that this model is associated with the biomedical disease model, as in that model the patient is just a body that needs fixing. Paternalism is predominantly viewed negatively in current medical practice, as the patient has no decision power or control. In extreme scenarios, this can lead to them being forced to undergo treatments and procedures to which they would not normally consent. That being said, paternalism is still part of medicine and is viewed as acceptable clinical practice. For example, in the United Kingdom, it is doctors who predominantly make decisions for neonates, not their parents; however, best practice is to involve parents and engage in the decision-making together (McGrath et al., 2021).

Some patients also prefer to defer to a healthcare professional's decision. In fact, in my own research on women who freeze reproductive tissue before undergoing harmful cancer treatments, many of the participants felt most comfortable making the choice to follow their doctor's decisions (Paton, 2017, 2018a, 2018b, 2019; Paton et al., 2020). They referred to this process as 'Being Guided' (Paton, 2019). Many of these women would have been more uncomfortable having to make many decisions throughout their treatment and instead wanted to be guided by the advice and simply comply with their doctor's chosen treatments (Paton, 2019). Taken at face value, this may appear to be paternalism, but in fact it is not. The crucial difference between being guided and true paternalism is that the patients choose to take this path: they choose to defer to the doctor's decision AND they can reverse that decision at any time. Paternalism does not offer the patient the chance to take back a decision they have made to give away control because that is not an option in the first place.

Mutuality

Mutuality is an interesting one. On paper it seems to tick all the boxes of what is expected in the modern clinical encounter. Mutuality is understood as a meeting between experts (Morgan, 2008). You've probably never heard of it, as research has shown that mutuality rarely occurs in practice (Morgan, 2008). It's not hard to see why. It is a highly idealised concept of the healthcare professional-patient relationship, which ignores the recognised embedded power of the healthcare professional in the clinical encounter. It assumes that all patients are knowledgeable about medicine, vocal about opinions and generally assertive. It is completely unrealistic, as it ignores all of the societal and cultural contexts surrounding medicine and health that we discussed in the earlier chapters. But it is one of the four types, so now you know—box ticked and all that.

Consumerism

Unsurprisingly, in this situation the patient is 'in control'. This takes us back to the beginnings of medicine, with a client-based approach. It is stereotypically seen as the relationship that must exist between healthcare professional and patient in fee-paying medical systems (e.g. the United States or private hospital model). However, again, this is not true in practice, as regardless of who is paying, the power dynamic always favours the healthcare professional to an extent (Paton, 2017).

A relationship of default

This is a model of the healthcare professional-patient relationship that has always puzzled me. The idea behind this model is that there apparently exist clueless patients with no direction or assertiveness AT ALL in their lives. They are simply floating through the world, passively giving way to everything. There is very little evidence of this in practice. More often, patients present as directionless when they are over-whelmed by information or lack an understanding of the situation. This means that, at best, a relationship of default may at times be present, but only until the patient has grasped the situation as best they can. This normally occurs due to poor com-munication between healthcare professionals and patients. A relationship of default can easily slide into paternalism if the healthcare professional is not self-aware about the situation.

Shared decision-making: solution or rhetoric?

So, what is actually happening between healthcare professionals and patients?

Patient involvement in decision-making is now viewed as the gold standard in clini-cal care (Paton et al., 2020). In the United Kingdom, this model dominates not just clinical practice but also policy and rhetoric (Paton et al., 2020). The approach is based on the principlist account of patient autonomy developed by Beauchamp and Childress (1994). Their account of autonomy prioritises informed understanding for the patient, by which they mean that the person making the decision should feel that they have suf-ficient information to be confident and comfortable that they understand the situation and are able to make decisions (Beauchamp and Childress, 1994; Paton et al., 2020). This informed understanding is achieved through non-directive counselling from the clinician, which provides the patient with information about the available options and then, ideally, supports the patient in making their own decision based on their prefer-ences, values and beliefs (Fried, 2016; Paton et al., 2020).

While shared decision-making makes a lot of sense—tell patients what the options are, give them any information they want on those options and then support the choice they make—this is not really what happens in practice (Fried, 2016; Paton et al., 2020). Instead, within the clinical encounter, healthcare professionals expect shared decision-making to look a particular 'way'; when it does not, the decisions patients make that fall outside of these expected norms can be viewed as 'wrong', 'unethical' or even 'irrational' by healthcare professionals (Paton et al., 2020). Spoiler alert—they are not.

As a result, even shared decision-making can reinforce unhelpful power relation-ships by suggesting that it is the healthcare professional who decides what is 'good' or 'ethical' decision-making for the patient, rather than the patient themselves. My own research on parents' decisions about whether to terminate a pregnancy after the prenatal diagnosis of a congenital anomaly serves as a helpful case study in under-standing the role that power plays in our perception of people's actions around their health.

In this research, we found that when parents made decisions in ways that did not conform to the expected style of shared decision-making that the doctors had learnt, the doctors viewed these decisions as irrational and even invalid in some way (Paton et al., 2020). This was especially true in the way parents interacted with clinical informa-tion to reach the state of informed understanding where they felt comfortable enough to make the decision. With all the groups in our study who wanted more, less or dif-ferent information from what their doctor had provided, their decisions were viewed as suspect by the doctor (Paton et al., 2020).

Just look at some of the things doctors said just because their patients wanted something different from what they had expected (a few words changed for anonymity reasons) (Paton et al., 2020):

> '[Clinicians] have got very much better at using words that are harder to Google. It makes a difference.'

> 'I have concerns that they really don't understand what they are going to let themselves in for. I mean if it's [information] available, why wouldn't you want to know?'

The study participants included religious parents who refused to terminate pregnancies for foetuses who would die in utero or shortly after birth, as their religious beliefs would not permit such a decision (Paton et al., 2020). This shows how important it is to understand the role that power and information have in the clinical encounter, as it is in fact rational and autonomous for someone to make a decision that is in line with their own belief systems. These are sound decisions that lead directly to health behaviours. Such decisions and behaviours were only viewed as irrational by doctors because the patients used non-clinical information to inform their decision.

By only accepting one 'way' of accessing and consuming information, the doctors in my study were stating that they not only knew better than the parents what information they needed but also the quantity of information and where it should come from (Paton et al., 2020). This reinforces the old-school, paternalistic view that the doctor STILL knows best, making them the more powerful member of the relationship. It is not an equal partnership, nor a facilitating one, as is understood in the discussion of shared decision-making. This highlights the need to improve our conception of what informed understanding really means and why different people will come to a point of informed understanding through different pathways, make decisions and behave accordingly (Paton et al., 2020).

Often, the way shared decision-making actually plays out in practice comes down to a battle between the concerns of the patient and the healthcare professionals' internalised views of their role and position. For example, 'old-school doctors' who follow a biomedical model will favour their expertise over the patient's expertise. Those who follow a holistic approach will view patient experiences as an important piece of the puzzle. It is effectively a crapshoot, dependent on the doctor in question. This is deeply problematic; not all models, as we have seen, are helpful in providing supportive healthcare. There is also a further layer of complexity, in that patients have internalised views of their role and position as a patient (Paton, 2017, 2018a, 2018b, 2019).

This means that it is still common to see a power dynamic that sets up the healthcare professional as the 'all-knowing' medical expert and the patient as the 'layperson'. Information is power in the clinical encounter, and the predominant models that favour medical knowledge over all other kinds mean that healthcare professionals are better equipped to translate that medical knowledge for patients, setting them up as the all-powerful keeper of information. The power dynamic is still strongly felt in the clinical encounter. While the paternalistic doctor is supposed to be a thing of the past, aspects still remain—not only in relation to informational power but also because class and educational differences are often vast in the clinical setting. Moreover, in the

United Kingdom in particular, there is a very strong sense that patients shouldn't be 'bothering' the very busy and important healthcare professionals, especially in the last few years with the NHS becoming increasingly busy and overwhelmed (Paton, 2017, 2018a, 2018b, 2019).

Conclusion

While, ultimately, people will do what they want to do, the different models and theories presented in this chapter represent a toolbox from which to pull useful and relevant models to support behaviour change in your patients and the wider population. Their influence is modest, but they can still help to support people looking to change their lifestyles and beliefs around health. As with every part of the body, context is the key. Interventions and support mechanisms that are out of sync with the context in which they operate will fail every time—leaving patients potentially worse off than when they started trying to change their behaviours. While behavioural change models are no silver bullet, when used mindfully they can provide the help and support needed to promote healthy living. However, the focus should not just be about what model might work best for a patient. The power dynamics within the healthcare professional-patient relationship influence the way information is accessed and consumed. While there have been some inroads towards a better understanding that every person makes decisions in different ways, there remain expectations from the clinical world that patients conform to certain approaches, which restrict patient autonomy and reinforce power dynamics that favour the healthcare professional over the patient.

Test Yourself

1. Define health-related behaviours.
2. Health-related behaviours that promote good health are known as:
   (a) Good habits
   (b) Positive health-protective behaviours
   (c) Low-risk behaviours
   (d) Health promotion
3. Pavlov discovered which theory of behaviour? Provide the name of the theory and a brief definition.
4. How does operant conditioning modify behaviour?
   (a) It modifies behaviour through reinforcement in the form of punishment or reward.
   (b) It modifies behaviour through positive association techniques.
   (c) It modifies behaviour through medication and counselling.
   (d) It modifies behaviour through negative association techniques.
5. What are the five different aspects of the Health Belief Model necessary to modify behaviour?

Note

1 Though, if you have children, you'll also know that who the reward chart 'rewards' or 'punishes', the child or the parent, changes on an almost daily basis.

References

Ajzen, I. (1991). 'The theory of planned behaviour.' *Organizational Behavior and Human Decision Processes* 50(2): 179–211. https://doi.org/10.1016/0749-5978(91)90020-T

APA (2018). 'Aversion conditioning.' *APA Dictionary of Psychology*. Available at: https://dictionary.apa.org/aversion-conditioning

Arno, A. and Thomas, S. (2016). 'The efficacy of nudge theory strategies in influencing adult dietary behaviour: A systematic review and meta-analysis.' *BMC Public Health* 16: 676. https://doi.org/10.1186/s12889-016-3272-x

Bandura, A. (1977). *Social learning theory.* Englewood Cliffs, NJ: Prentice-Hall Inc.

Beauchamp, T.L. and Childress, J.F. (1994). *Principles of biomedical ethics.* Edicoes Loyola.

CMS (n.d.). 'Chemical aversion therapy for treatment of alcoholism.' *Medicare Coverage Database*. Available at: https://www.cms.gov/medicare-coverage-database/view/ncd.aspx?NCDId=30&ncdver=1

Davison, K., Hubbard, K., Marks, S., Spandler, H. and Wynter, R. (2024). 'An inclusive history of LGBTQ+ aversion therapy: Past harms and future address in a UK context.' *Review of General Psychology* 29(1): 33–48. https://doi.org/10.1177/10892680241289904

Faries, M.D. (2016). 'Why we don't "Just Do It": Understanding the intention-behavior gap in lifestyle medicine.' *American Journal of Lifestyle Medicine* 10(5): 322–329. https://doi.org/10.1177/1559827616638017

Festinger, L. (1957). *A theory of cognitive dissonance.* Stanford: Stanford University Press.

Fried, T.R. (2016). 'Shared decision making—Finding the sweet spot.' *New England Journal of Medicine* 374(2): 104–106. https://doi.org/10.1056/NEJMp1510020

Gibbons, S.M., Schwartz, T., Fouquier, J., Mitchell, M., Sangwan, N., Gilbert, J.A. and Kelley, S.T. (2015). 'Ecological succession and viability of human-associated microbiota on restroom surfaces.' *Applied and Environmental Microbiology* 81(2): 765–773. https://doi.org/10.1128/AEM.03117-14

Hagger, M.S., Chan, D.K.C., Protogerou, C. and Chatzisarantis, N.L.D. (2016). 'Using meta-analytic path analysis to test theoretical predictions in health behavior: An illustration based on meta-analyses of the theory of planned behavior.' *Preventative Medicine* 89: 154–161. https://doi.org/10.1016/j.ypmed.2016.05.020

Hagger, M.S. and Hamilton, K. (2021). 'Effects of socio-structural variables in the theory of planned behavior: A mediation model in multiple samples and behaviors.' *Psychology & Health* 36(3): 307–333. https://doi.org/10.1080/08870446.2020.1784420

Hochbaum, G., Rosentock, I. and Kegek, S. (1952). *Health belief model.* US Public Health Service.

McCabe, B. (2014). 'Hopkins researcher discovers everything we know about Pavlov is wrong.' *Johns Hopkins Magazine*. Available at: https://hub.jhu.edu/magazine/2014/winter/daniel-todes-biography-of-pavlov/ [accessed 21st January 2025].

McGrath, J., Vasu, V. and Sullivan, C. (2021). 'Shared decision making: Translating guidance into practice.' *Infant* 17(4): 146–149. Available at: https://www.infantjournal.co.uk/pdf/inf_100_7229.pdf

Meikle, J. (2015). 'Almost one in four deaths "avoidable with lifestyle and healthcare changes".' *The Guardian*, 20th May. Available at: https://www.theguardian.com/uk-news/2015/may/20/deaths-avoidable-lifestyle-healthcare-england-wales-ons

Michie, S., van Stralen, M. and West, R. (2011). 'The behaviour change wheel: A new method for characterising and designing behaviour change interventions.' *BMC Implementation Science* 6: 42. https://doi.org/10.1186/1748-5908-6-42

Michie, S., West, R., Pidgeon, N., Reicher, S., Amlôt, R. and Bear, L. (2021). 'Staying "Covid-safe": Proposals for embedding behaviours that protect against Covid-19 transmission in the UK.' *British Journal of Health Psychology* 26(4): 1238–1257. https://doi.org/10.1111/bjhp.12557

Minton, H.L. (2002). *Departing from deviance: A history of homosexual rights and emancipatory science in America.* University of Chicago Press.

Morgan, M. (2008). 'The doctor-patient relationship.' In *Sociology as applied to health* [6th Edition], edited by G. Scambler (pp. 55–70). London: Saunders Elsevier.

NHS (n.d.). *Quit smoking*. Available at: https://www.nhs.uk/better-health/quit-smoking/

NICE (2014). *Behaviour change: Individual approaches*. Available at: https://www.nice.org.uk/guidance/ph49

Office for National Statistics (2024). *Avoidable mortality in England and Wales: 2021 and 2022*. Available at: https://www.ons.gov.uk/peoplepopulationandcommunity/healthandsocialcare/causesofdeath/bulletins/avoidablemortalityinenglandandwales/2021and2022

Paton, A. (2017). 'No Longer Handmaiden: The role of social and sociological theory in bioethics.' *International Journal of Feminist Approaches to Bioethics* 10(1): 30–49. https://doi.org/10.3138/ijfab.10.1.30

Paton, A. (2018a). 'About time: How time influences and facilitates patient autonomy in the clinical encounter.' *Monash Bioethics Review* 36: 68–85. https://doi.org/10.1007/s40592-018-0089-7

Paton, A. (2018b). '"It's not just about having babies": A socio-bioethical exploration of older women's experiences of making oncofertility decisions in Britain.' In *Philosophies and sociologies of bioethics*, edited by H. Riesch, N. Emmerich and S. Wainwright. Springer.

Paton, A. (2019). '"Being Guided": What oncofertility patients' decisions can teach us about the efficacy of autonomy, agency and decision-making theory in the contemporary clinical encounter.' *International Journal of Feminist Approaches to Bioethics* 12(2): 18–35. https://doi.org/10.3138/ijfab.12.2.02

Paton, A., Armstrong, N., Smith, L. and Lotto, R. (2020). 'Parents' decision-making following diagnosis of a severe congenital anomaly in pregnancy: Practical, theoretical and ethical tensions.' *Social Science and Medicine* 266: 113362. https://doi.org/10.1016/j.socscimed.2020.113362

Prochaska, J.O. and DiClemente, C.C. (1983). 'Stages and processes of self-change of smoking: Toward an integrative model of change.' *Journal of Consulting and Clinical Psychology* 51(3): 390–395. https://doi.org/10.1037/0022-006X.51.3.390

Silverman, K. (2004). 'Exploring the limits and utility of operant conditioning in the treatment of drug addiction.' *Behavior Analyst* 27(2): 209–230. https://doi.org/10.1007/BF03393181

Skinner, B.F. (1937). 'Two types of conditioned reflex: A reply to Konorski and Miller.' *Journal of General Psychology* 16(1): 272–279. http://dx.doi.org/10.1080/00221309.1937.9917951

Skinner, B.F. (1963). 'Operant behavior.' *American Psychologist* 18(8): 503–515. https://doi.org/10.1037/h0045185

Thaler, R. and Sustein, C. (2008). *Nudge: Improving decisions about health, wealth and happiness*. New Haven: Yale University Press.

Thrailkill, E.A. and Rey, C.N. (2024). 'Pavlovian conditioning: Principles to guide application.' In *Behavior analysis: Translational perspectives and clinical practice*, edited by H.S. Roane, A.R. Craig, V. Saini and J.E. Ringdahl (pp. 123–145). The Guilford Press.

UKParliament (2020). 'Rapid response. COVID-19: Behavioural and social interventions.' *POST*, 26th March. Available at: https://post.parliament.uk/covid-19-behavioural-and-social-interventions/ [accessed 4th March 2025].

West, R. (2007). *Theory of addiction*. Oxford: Wiley Blackwell.

West, R. and Brown, J. (2013). *Theory of addiction*. John Wiley and Sons.

Wethington, E., Glanz, K. and Schwartz, M.D. (2015). 'Stress, coping, and health behavior.' In *Health behavior: Theory, research, and practice* [5th Edition], edited by K. Glanz, B.K. Rimer and K. Viswanath (pp. 223–242). Jossey-Bass.

Woolf, S.H. and Aron, L. (eds.) (2013). *U.S. health in international perspective: Shorter lives, poorer health*. Washington, DC: National Academies Press. Available at: https://www.ncbi.nlm.nih.gov/books/NBK154472/

World Health Organisation (n.d.). *Indicator metadata registry list*. Available at: https://www.who.int/data/gho/indicator-metadata-registry/imr-details/3419

CHAPTER 5

Promoting health and wellbeing

Understanding how people develop health beliefs, which translate into their willingness to be healthy, is an important part of understanding your patients' health. Promoting health and wellbeing at the individual and population levels requires you, as their healthcare professional, to understand how to tailor your approach and relationship with patients to best support them in engaging with the treatment best suited to their lifestyles and beliefs.

This chapter will cover these concepts at the individual and population level. At the individual level, we will cover three core concepts: adherence, concordance and patient-centredness. At the population level we will delve into public health, looking at the way health promotion and screening programmes support (or fail to support) overall population health and wellbeing.

Adherence

In healthcare, when advice is followed, it is called adherence. This was originally called compliance, but the paternalistic elements of insisting that patients 'comply' with their healthcare professional's advice or treatment plans is at odds with modern healthcare and its goals of patient-centred care. Over time, the term 'compliance' became viewed as limiting and stigmatizing for the patient—especially for people with long-term conditions. The WHO instead adopted the term 'adherence', defining it as:

> [T]he extent to which a patient's medication-taking behaviour and/or execution of lifestyle changes corresponds with agreed recommendations from a healthcare provider.
>
> *(Sabaté, 2003)*

Adherence is an important concept in healthcare because it is not only about persuading patients to follow healthcare professionals' advice; there are also known and proven

DOI: 10.4324/9781032677552-5

benefits. In simple terms, the more someone adheres to a treatment, the better the clinical outcomes for their issue or condition. However, people don't always adhere to their treatments. Adherence is most often discussed with regards to medication, so let's look at the numbers there first.

When someone does not adhere, it is called non-adherence. Non-adherence does not necessarily mean that someone is not taking ANY of their medication—just that they are not taking it as directed. This is pretty common. In a study carried out a few years ago, it was found that between 20% and 30% of patients do not take their medication as prescribed (van Dulmen et al., 2007). Sometimes this is referred to as secondary non-adherence—which, of course, might have you asking 'if that is secondary, then what is primary?' Fear not. I've got your back.

While most non-adherence involves some sort of engagement with the medication or treatment prescribed, patients not taking medication at all is still a significant problem in healthcare. About 17% of people never pick up their prescriptions—a phenomenon known as primary non-adherence (Zeitouny et al., 2023). Interestingly, in a study that looked at the prescription habits of around 34,000 patients, older patients were much more likely to pick up their prescriptions then younger patients. However, once patients were over the age of 65 and had more than one prescription to fill and pick up, the rates of primary non-adherence increased (Zeitouny et al., 2023).

This study pinpoints a flaw early on in our discussion about adherence that is worth thinking through. On the face of it, people should want to adhere to treatment because it will improve clinical outcomes—who doesn't want to feel better? However, life is never that simple: either improved clinical outcomes are not an incentive or priority, or, as the research above illustrates, the desire to adhere can be there but the ability to adhere may be lacking. For example, as people age, it can be harder to make repeated trips to the pharmacy. The will is there, but the ability just isn't. Of course, adherence relates to more than just medication. It applies to all sorts of treatments and therapies—diet and lifestyle changes, physiotherapy, counselling. All of these can be difficult for people for a wide variety of reasons.

Non-adherence is almost more important a concept than adherence because non-adherence does not just lead to poorer health outcomes for the individual—it has huge costs for the whole healthcare system. In England alone, the cost of non-adherence, measured in health lost, was estimated 15 years ago to be about £500 million annually (York Health Economics Consortium, 2010). Accounting for inflation, that is just under £760 million per year in 2025 (Bank of England, 2025). This was caused by an estimated £300 million (at the time) in wasted medicine annually (York Health Economics Consortium, 2010). Again, this amounts to around £530 million in today's money (Bank of England, 2025).

Sure, £760 million is only 0.4% of the overall NHS budget for England (£179 billion in the 2024–2025 fiscal year) (Arnold and Jefferies, 2025), but when you consider that it is almost enough to run a large NHS trust such as the one in Coventry for a year, you start to get an idea of just how that money could be used (AdLife, n.d.). I am sharing these figures not to shame patients who do not adhere to treatments, but to show the sheer scale of non-adherence and why it is so important as healthcare professionals to try and understand why patients take this path and how to support them, leaving them in a better position to adhere to treatment plans. More on that shortly.

Concordance

It would seem logical that if the goal is to persuade a patient to adhere to a recommended treatment, some sort of agreement should be reached that supports this adherence. This is where we often hear the term concordance. Concordance occurs when a patient and healthcare professional agree on the best treatment plan for the patient (Aronson, 2007). The idea is that people can and should be involved in their own care; when they are, they are more likely to adhere to their treatment plan.

Like so many concepts where healthcare professionals and patients work together, the concept of concordance carries several assumptions that make it likely more of an ideal then a reality. For example, it assumes people should and can speak as equals to their healthcare professionals—something that, as we know from the previous chapter, can be difficult to achieve given the existing power dynamics between healthcare professionals and patients. It also assumes that all patients want more involvement in their treatment decisions. Again, as we saw with my own work on 'Being Guided', this is not everyone's preference (Paton, 2019). Many patients, for a variety of reasons, do not want to take on responsibility for their treatment plan themselves.

However, despite these drawbacks, the concept of concordance at least nods to the autonomy and agency of patients. Concordance opens the door for the health behaviour field to consider the benefits of working with patients more widely to develop the best treatment plans for them—which may not be the best clinical choice, but one the patient can at least consistently follow. Ultimately, the extent to which a patient adheres (or doesn't) to a treatment plan is more of a continuum than a binary relationship. People tend to adhere to a greater or lesser extent to treatment; it is less common to have a patient who does not adhere to any aspect of a treatment at all.

There are two recognised reasons for non-adherence. The first is intentional non-adherence. Intentional non-adherence is fairly self-evident: the patient intentionally, that is on purpose, does not follow the prescribed treatment (Usherwood, 2017). Intentional non-adherence is most often due to the patient's beliefs about the recommended treatment and whether it will be effective or necessary to undergo that treatment plan.

The second reason is unintentional non-adherence. This occurs when a patient's non-adherence to a treatment is not a deliberate act. Instead, they are not adhering due to forgetfulness, difficulty accessing certain medicines/therapies or misunderstanding how to engage with the treatment plan correctly (Usherwood, 2017).

Again, understanding why your patient is not sticking to a treatment plan is important, as adherence will lead to better health outcomes for the patient. While people can be more or less adherent, there is a sweet spot where a certain level of adherence improves health outcomes. A study from 2018 found that there needs to be an adherence rate of at least 80% for a patient to achieve the best health outcomes for their treatment plan (Kim et al., 2018). Given this sweet spot for adherence, it is in everybody's best interests to work with patients to help them adhere as best they can to treatment plans.

Improving adherence: the multidimensional model

Improving adherence is so important that, a little over 20 years ago, the WHO developed a model to help better understand the influences on adherence. The Multidimensional

Model identifies five key factors important in adherence that help us understand how complex adherence really is (Sabaté, 2003):

1. Disease or condition-related factors

People are more likely to adhere to treatment if they are experiencing illness symptoms. This is because they want the symptoms to go away and following the treatment is seen as a way to achieve this goal. This is why antibiotics packaging always tells the recipient to finish the course of treatment even if they start to feel better: as symptoms diminish, people are less likely to adhere to treatment pathways, as they perceive themselves as feeling better.

2. Treatment or therapy-related factors

This is a simple relationship—the more difficult a treatment is to follow consistently, the less the patient will adhere to it. This difficulty can be linked to side effects or the need for changes in lifestyle or behaviours, or just the complexity (such as needing to take a medicine at a particular time of day).

3. Patient-related factors

Motivation is the key to this factor. As we saw in a previous chapter, patients must see the benefits of a treatment in order to be motivated to engage in that treatment. The seriousness of the illness, as perceived by the patient, also serves as motivation for adherence. Of course, there should also be minimal barriers to following the treatment. All of these, brought together, influence the overall motivation of the patient to adhere. The Patient-Related Factors in the Multidimensional Model are very similar to the Health Belief Model we covered in the previous chapter. As you can already see, these three factors do not stand on their own; they are strongly interconnected. Severity of illness and complexity of treatment can easily influence a person's motivation to adhere to a treatment. A strength of the Multidimensional Model is that it is able to bring together the complex ways in which the world around us impacts the decisions and actions that we make for our health.

4. Social and economic factors

Here, I need you to remember everything from the chapter on the social determinants of health and the influence they have on people's actions and beliefs about their health. The influence they have on adherence is very similar. For example, people with better support networks are more likely to adhere to their treatment. Equally, poverty and deprivation can negatively impact adherence—not only because people lack the financial resources to access a medication or therapy but also due to less obvious barriers such as being unable to afford transport to a clinic or pharmacy. Social, cultural and religious beliefs can also preclude people from engaging in certain treatment pathways. Race is another factor that impacts on adherence; for example, due to the appalling history of being used for human experimentation, Black communities are often more mistrusting of medical professionals and thus less likely to adhere to treatment pathways

(Sabaté, 2003; Benoit et al., 2023). When you consider such atrocities as the Tuskegee syphilis scandal,[1] you can understand why some communities are naturally cautious when told something is clinically 'good' for them by a group of professionals who have not historically had their best interests at heart (McVean, 2019).

5.   Health systems and healthcare team factors

Healthcare is a two-way street. It is not just the patient's responsibility to adhere to the treatment; the healthcare system itself must do its best to facilitate that adherence. First, there are of course practical issues with adherence. Does the patient have easy access to healthcare services? What are the costs of the services—not only financial costs but also such things as wait times? These factors are often overlooked in policies around adherence, but the ease of use of a system plays a big part in whether a patient can actually adhere to a treatment. In my own work in the deprived neighbourhoods of Birmingham, residents reported constant difficulties in accessing healthcare services such as diabetes clinics, physiotherapy and paediatric mental health services. These were services they needed to access in order to adhere to their various treatment pathways, but the services had been cut by the local authority over time and never replaced (Benoit et al., 2023). As a result, only people who could either afford to pay for private care or to travel to a neighbourhood that did have those services were actually able to adhere to their treatment pathways (Benoit et al., 2023). These patients badly wanted to adhere to the treatment they were prescribed, but the healthcare system itself got in the way.

In addition to the healthcare system itself, the healthcare team plays a vital part in facilitating adherence for patients. Recall our previous discussion of the important role the healthcare professional-patient relationship plays in healthcare. The tone of that relationship, in particular the level of trust and empathy that the patient feels in the relationship, is key in whether a patient will adhere to treatment (Sabaté, 2003). In brief, the more heard and understood a patient feels, the more comfortable they will be in asking the healthcare professional for the information they need to understand their clinical situation. All of this makes it more likely that the patient will decide to adhere to the treatment. This creates a therapeutic alliance between the patient and healthcare professional that is recognised as a key part of facilitating adherence (Stubbe, 2018).

So now we know what influences adherence, but how do we improve it? With so many factors influencing adherence it can seem daunting to try and improve it at all; however, there are a number of ways to do so. Some are very simple, such as the reminder text messages patients receive to attend a clinical appointment or pick up a prescription from a pharmacy. Educating patients about the importance of adherence also leads to improvements. Methods can also be more hands-on, such as speaking to patients about planning their lives so as to improve adherence to a particular treatment—something known as motivational interviewing (Aronson, 2007). It will come as no surprise that, for something that can be explained via a 'multidimensional' model, the solutions are also multidimensional. The most successful approach to improving adherence is to tackle several issues at once, as providing a solution for only one factor does not properly address the interconnectedness of the key factors of adherence for patients (Aronson, 2007).

Practitioner-Patient Communication (P-P Communication)

Most non-adherence boils down to a problem in communication between the patient and practitioner. Poor communication can mean, for example, that a patient's concerns about a treatment plan are not properly heard or understood by their healthcare professional. As a result, these concerns are not addressed and the patient doesn't adhere to the plan because—well, why would they if they have worries about it? One possible solution to this is Practitioner-Patient Communication, more commonly known as P-P Communication.

P-P Communication is not just about speaking effectively with a patient. It emphasises the importance of non-verbal and verbal communication in showing understanding, empathy and respect to the patient (Street Jr et al., 2009). P-P Communication recognises that a patient-centred approach is the most effective medicine (Street Jr et al., 2009). As we saw in our discussion of power in the healthcare professional-patient relationship, there is a clinician agenda and a patient agenda in the clinical encounter. These don't always match up (because people are different!). P-P Communication is a way to bring these two agendas together, aligning them in a way that promotes trust and respect between the patient and healthcare professional (Street Jr et al., 2009). The result? Better adherence to the agreed treatment. It is amazing what some respect, empathy and trust can do. Remember that.

The principles of P-P Communication
There are four key elements necessary for P-P Communication (Scales et al., 2003):

1.   Develop Discrepancy

This element of P-P Communication involves explaining to patients that their current actions/behaviours are not aligned with their future goals. This part of the conversation is non-judgemental. The goal is to give the patient the space to consider what their goals are, raise concerns they have and ultimately support the patient in resetting their health goals.

2.   Avoid Argumentation

Helping people see the discrepancies in their behaviour can be challenging. People don't like confronting the reality that they may have been going about something in the wrong way or have misunderstood something. Defensiveness is natural, but a key element of P-P Communication is avoiding an argument. Doing this builds trust and shows understanding. You, as the healthcare professional, need to embrace the resistance and try and help the patient to see and understand their situation from a different point of view. Doing so helps the patient fully grasp why their health goals and health behaviours are leading to non-adherence.

What this really means is that the role of the healthcare professional is to help patients break down what they need to do. How many of us put off big tasks because they are daunting or overwhelming? Most of us. In fact, I'm writing this very chapter in my unfinished garden because it turns out laying a patio when you've never done one before is pretty daunting AND overwhelming. But a plan of small, simple steps can help. I can dig out the space one day. Level the space the next. Fill in the hole with hardcore in two weeks' time. Slowly, the patio gets done. Small and simple steps will eventually get me where I need to go. The same principle applies here.

3.   Roll with Resistance

P-P Communication is not only about how we share information with each other in the clinical encounter but also about emotions felt in that encounter. We already know that everyone has beliefs about health that guide their actions. It is important to roll with any resistance to change and take the opportunity to discuss why that resistance is there in the first place. People don't like to be ordered to do things or to be imposed upon—just ask my toddler when I'm trying to get her to wear pants. The goal is instead to support the patient, facilitating conversation and reflection that helps the patient challenge their own resistance and emotions. Doing so will help them find the belief in themselves and the resources they need to adhere to the treatment or change.

4.   Express Empathy

Empathy is probably one of the most important clinical skills you will need when working in healthcare. People want and need to feel understood. Empathy—true empathy, I will add—with your patients can help many of them to accept the necessary changes that will improve their health. Reflective listening is key to this because it builds trust and indicates to your patient that you are really listening to them—their concerns, their questions and their fears.

A quick guide to reflective listening

Reflective listening is a great technique to use in your practice. It helps your patient feel valued and respected and helps you to learn about their needs. The #1 rule with reflective listening is that it isn't about you. It really isn't. Park your needs and ego and everything else at the door. When practising medicine and working in healthcare, the focus is often on what you can do for the patient. However, with reflective listening, you aren't trying to figure out what you can do for your patient, but what they can do for themselves (Buffington et al., 2016). The goal of reflective listening is to help you and your patient understand how they view and understand themselves.

Reflective listening is largely done using mirroring and paraphrasing (Stein and Hurd, 2000).

Mirroring involves repeating back key phrases said by the speaker. They might say: 'I'm really frustrated that I lost my car keys and missed my train to work'.

When mirroring you would reply: 'You lost your car keys and missed your train'.

Paraphrasing is repeating back to the speaker a rephrased version of what they said. If we use the same example as above, you might reply: 'You're frustrated because that made you late for work'.

You'll know you are doing active listening 'right' if (Stein and Hurd, 2000):

■   You listen more than you talk
■   You haven't asked questions

- You focus on restating and clarifying what has been said
- You don't say what you feel, but keep the frame of reference on the patient

Public and population health

The first half of this chapter has focused on promoting good health for individuals, but good health at a population level is just as important. Population and public health refers to the overall health of groups, communities and populations. Unlike individual health, public health takes a broader focus, seeking to promote good health through education, awareness and prevention. Many of the concepts used in public health draw from health behaviour theory and models, but are applied to groups. In the second half of this chapter we examine different public health strategies, types of prevention and some of the issues with existing public health approaches.

What is public health?

There are three main domains of public health: health protection, health improvement and health service delivery. They all interact with each other (Faculty of Public Health, 2025) (Figure 5.1).

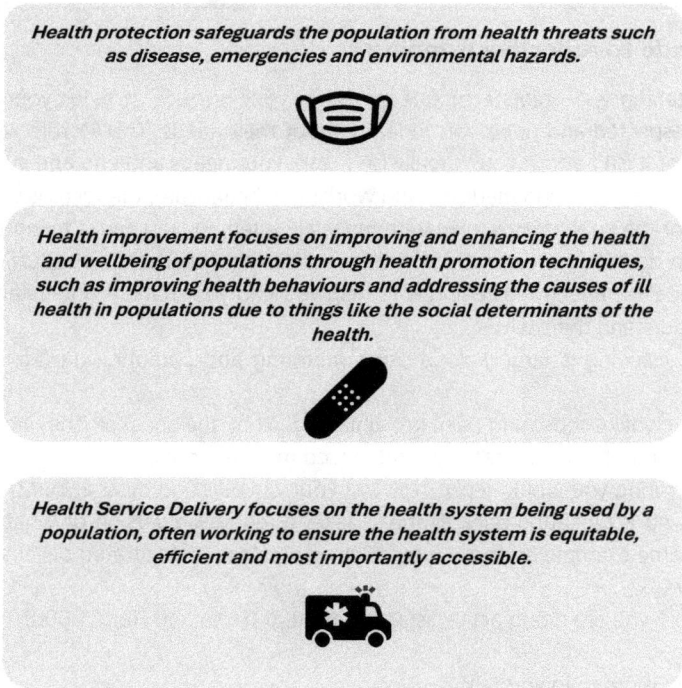

Health protection safeguards the population from health threats such as disease, emergencies and environmental hazards.

Health improvement focuses on improving and enhancing the health and wellbeing of populations through health promotion techniques, such as improving health behaviours and addressing the causes of ill health in populations due to things like the social determinants of the health.

Health Service Delivery focuses on the health system being used by a population, often working to ensure the health system is equitable, efficient and most importantly accessible.

Figure 5.1 The Three Main Domains of Public Health.

Prevention is better than cure

You'll remember from earlier chapters that we are living longer than ever before, but that life is lived with more illness these days. However, we needn't be condemned to a long life of ill health. In fact, research has shown that for heart disease, which is one of the biggest killers in society, preventative care would actually prevent or postpone a third of such deaths (Kottke et al., 2009).

We have a lot of incentive to prevent ill health beyond simply not dying. Good health results in a more productive and stronger economy, while reducing pressures on vital health and social care services (Department of Health and Social Care, 2018). Ultimately, a focus on prevention of ill health also creates a more sustainable health system that is better prepared to care for future generations. Not to get all heavy, but prevention is key to both population wellbeing and healthcare system survival. As a result, there has been considerable work over the years to prevent ill health at the population level.

The four levels of prevention

So, we know prevention is important, but what actions can be taken and what does prevention 'look' like in practice? There are four levels of prevention in public health (Kisling and Das, 2023). Let's look at each of these now.

Primordial prevention

Primordial prevention strategies aim to improve health and prevent ill health by targeting the social and environmental conditions that bring about ill health in the first place. They are designed to tackle the social determinants of health at source, changing policies, regulations and laws that negatively impact health. Primordial prevention often targets childhood health, as the earlier in the life course the prevention, the better. Kisling and Das use the example of changing policies to improve pavements; this is a good way of understanding how broad primordial prevention activities can be. On the face of it, it is hard to see how improving the quality and availability of pavements in a community would have much impact on health, but it is a small, environmental change that can lead to a significant health improvement for the population. Better pavements mean that people are more likely to walk. This increases their physical activity, which has positive knock-on effects, reducing risk factors for diseases such as obesity and Type 2 diabetes (Kisling and Das, 2023). In this way, primordial prevention doesn't always relate to changing health policy, but instead to achieving a wider, seemingly unrelated change with positive consequences for the health of the population.

Primary prevention

The aim of primary prevention is to prevent disease or injury from occurring by reducing the risk factors for those diseases and injuries. Most of us have engaged in primary prevention activities since childhood through classic examples such as immunisation. The idea behind primary prevention is that if disease and injury are prevented from occurring then the population (and the health services) don't need to deal with more complex advanced disease later on. This is better, overall, for the health of the population. Health promotion campaigns are another good example of a primary prevention activity. There are several that many of you will find familiar: for example the 5-a-day campaign in the United Kingdom, created to increase fruit and vegetable consumption, is a classic example of a health promotion campaign aiming to reduce obesity and improve health. More recently, campaigns to protect against the flu, such as the slogan 'Catch it. Bin it. Kill it.', have been carried out to reduce the spread of infectious disease (Department of Health and Social Care, 2013).

Secondary prevention

While the first two forms of prevention aim to prevent disease and injury before it can even begin, secondary prevention recognises that not all ill health can be avoided. The goal of secondary prevention is to detect and treat disease or risk factors at an early stage, often before symptoms even appear. It is well recognised that earlier intervention is more effective and successful, making it more likely that disease progression can be slowed or even stopped. Screening programmes, which look for early signs or risk factors of diseases such as cancer, are a good example of secondary prevention activities. Routine monitoring of risk factors such as blood pressure and blood sugar levels are other examples of secondary prevention activities designed to 'catch' disease early. While not very exciting, or all that interesting for many, these kinds of consistent, routine tests can make a huge life-or-death difference (UK National Screening Committee, 2025).

Tertiary prevention

Finally, tertiary prevention is the final barricade in trying to prevent ill health in the population. Tertiary prevention focuses on minimising the effects and impact of established disease. Tertiary prevention activities can be small, everyday activities such as using steroids to prevent asthma attacks. They can also be complex, such as organ transplant to treat failing organs like the kidney or heart due to disease. With tertiary prevention, the horse has already bolted, so the focus is on minimising the damage and ideally stopping further ill health in the future.

Health promotion

Much of the health and wellbeing promotion in the population takes place via primary and secondary prevention activities. For the rest of this chapter, we are going to focus on the two most common forms of this prevention: health promotion and screening.

Health promotion was defined by the Ottawa Charter for Health Promotion in 1986 as 'The process of enabling people to increase control over and to improve their health' (World Health Organisation, 1986). Health promotion strategies focus largely on education and awareness. The Ottawa Charter set out six key aspects of health promotion that should inform all health promotion activities:

1. Building healthy public policy: this is very much a nod to primordial prevention and the important role that public policy plays at the population level.
2. Creating supportive environments: while we often think of physical and mental health when discussing public health and health promotion, the role played by the natural and built environment in promoting health (or not) is an important part of overall population health.

3. Strengthening community action: this aspect of health promotion emphasises the importance of empowering and enabling communities to access opportunities for better health.
4. Developing personal skills: education is essential to most health promotion strategies, as it allows people and populations to learn about options and choices for healthier lives, thus enabling healthy choices and giving people the skills and information to take control of their health.
5. Re-orientating health services: health services can be a key part of health promotion by helping provide the kind of education, information and health services required to support good health more holistically.
6. Moving into the future: ultimately, health promotion views good health as an investment worth making. Health promotion can help promote better health equity as well as improvements to the wider socio-ecological determinants of health.

Types of health promotion
As the aim of health promotion is to improve the health of as many people as possible, it can be targeted or universal. Universal approaches aim to improve health and reduce risk across a whole population. A good example of universal health promotion is the so-called 'sugar tax' in the United Kingdom. Universal approaches work well where a risk factor is common, as it will have a bigger overall impact. However, this is not without its disadvantages: there is a risk, with universal approaches to health promotion, of the harm paradox. When the population risk is high, but the individual risk is low for many, the harm paradox occurs because some people do not perceive the health 'threat' as relevant to themselves, leading to a lower uptake of the promoted action or behaviour.

'Sugar taxes': do they work?

Brought in to reduce sugar intake in the UK population, and specifically to target rising childhood obesity rates, the Soft Drink Industry Levy was introduced by the UK government in April 2018 (HM Treasury, 2018). More commonly called the 'Sugar Tax', the levy resulted in over half of manufacturers reducing sugar in their drinks before it even came into effect (HM Treasury, 2018). In 2018, this equated to a removal of about 45 million kilograms of sugar from the market per year. For those of you, like me, who don't enjoy sugary drinks, that is the equivalent of 957,446,808 Reese's Peanut Butter Cups going uneaten in a year. Unfortunately, I've likely destroyed the statistics for 2025 by consuming them in the thousands while writing this book.

Despite my peanut butter and chocolate relapse, the sugar tax has been a success. It is thought to have prevented around 40,000 cases of obesity in primary school-aged girls and has significantly improved dental hygiene since its introduction (Thomas, 2024).

Targeted approaches to health promotion are aimed at specific, at-risk populations or specific risk behaviour. The benefit is that they can be tailored to the needs of these particular populations or communities. However, as with universal approaches, caution is needed. Targeted approaches to health promotion risk falling into the assumption that groups are homogenous. This, in turn, can lead to health issues being neglected if they are not believed to occur in a particular community. In worse cases, it can lead to culture blaming, whereby poor health is lazily blamed on a community's cultural beliefs or attitudes towards a health issue. When this happens, the wider causes of ill health for that community may be ignored in favour of targeting specific behaviours or beliefs instead of working with communities to improve health more broadly. A good example of a targeted health promotion campaign is the series of smoking cessation campaigns that have run in the United Kingdom for several years now.

Regardless of whether the approach is universal or tailored, there are five established ways of 'doing' health promotion (Ewles and Simnett, 2003). Let's consider them from the point of view of smoking cessation:

1. Medical: medical health promotion uses clinical interventions to prevent and improve ill health. This could include medication to assist with smoking cessation or screening for lung cancer in current and ex-smokers.
2. Behaviour change: this type of health promotion uses the theories discussed in the previous chapter to support smokers in changing their health behaviours and reduce risky behaviour. One example are those apps discussed earlier that tell smokers how much money they are saving by not smoking, thus showing them a reward for better health behaviour.
3. Educational: this approach to health promotion does what it says on the tin. The focus is on providing information to give people a knowledge and understanding about health that enable them to make healthier choices and actions. Awareness campaigns about the risks of smoking are a good example.
4. Empowerment: sometimes called the client-centred approach, empowerment provides people with the knowledge and skills they need to improve their health; this can include smoking cessation courses and apps.
5. Societal change: this final approach focuses on improving and changing the physical and social environment that influences health. In the case of smoking, smoking bans in public places, such as restaurants, are a good example of this type of health promotion.

Screening

We've now covered prevention and promotion, but I want to take a more in-depth look at screening, as it is a form of secondary prevention—identifying disease or pre-disease states at an early stage—that has also developed into a form of health promotion, as it has made people aware of diseases that need screening and also boosted diagnosis for these diseases. In large part, the purpose of screening for diseases/conditions is to provide a better outcome than when something is found in the usual way—that is the patient has symptoms and self-reports to health services when these symptoms become burdensome. We don't screen for conditions where treatment can wait until there are symptoms. Instead, the aim is, for the most part, early detection of diseases where diagnosis at an early stage in its progression will lead to a better prognosis (outcome) for the patient.

Again, as with health promotion, screening programmes will be familiar to you, and many of you will have already participated in at least one (UK Government, n.d.a). For example, as a woman under 40 who has had children, I have had cervical screening and also foetal anomaly screening when I was pregnant; my children have had a NIPE (Newborn and Infant Physical Examination), a blood spot and a hearing screening. Screening is a regular part of our 'medical life' and will be a regular feature in your practice too.

What is screening?

Screening, at its most basic, is to identify whether further diagnostic tests are needed. Often, a rapid test determines whether someone is at high or low risk of the disease. The person is labelled as 'screen positive' or 'screen negative' based on the results of the test. This does not mean that they *definitely* have the disease; it just means they are at high risk. The screening test helps identify who needs further tests to enable a diagnosis of disease. Treatment will only follow once a definitive diagnosis is made and if a treatment is possible (Figure 5.2).

While screening programmes are aimed at creating a healthier population, there are advantages and disadvantages to screening. Screening 'turns' otherwise healthy people into patients. This is a transformation that is not without consequences. Some argue that screening for a disease that cannot be altered, managed or cured may be an unethical practice, as all it does is satisfy a medical curiosity, while offering no benefit to the patient (Cochrane and Holland, 1971). In the United Kingdom, to help prevent over-use of screening and the potential harms that could result, there are five criteria for what should be screened and how they are used (UK National Screening Committee, 2022): Condition, Test, Intervention, Screening Programme and Implementation (Wilson and Jungner, 1968). Let's look at each of these now, as it will help shape our understanding of why some conditions that seem like good candidates for screening currently have no screening programme.

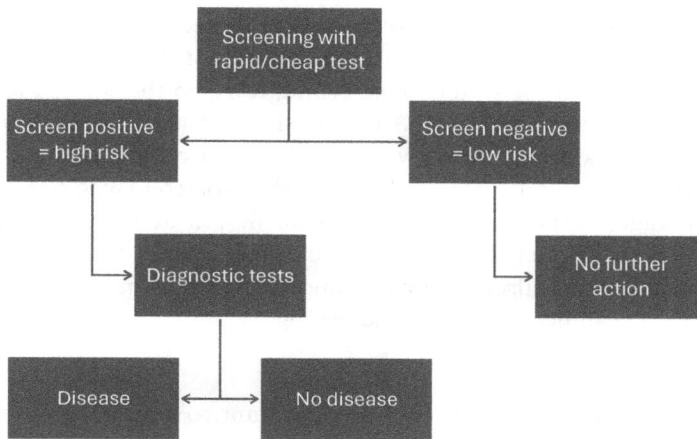

Figure 5.2 Flowchart of the Process of Basic Screening Programmes.

1. Condition

Normally, conditions are screened if they are considered to be a health problem of significant frequency or severity. The prevalence, incidence and natural history of the disease must also be well understood. In general, it should be a serious disease where we have a good knowledge of how it is spread and the impact it has on the population. All possible primary interventions, such as immunisations, behaviours and measures to reduce infection, must already have been put into practice as far as is possible—meaning that all possible attempts to reduce the likelihood of someone actually getting the disease have been made. Importantly, the psychological implications of diagnosis for the patient should also be considered. This is especially important for genetic mutations that cause disease, or hereditary disease, and relates to the previously mentioned concerns about the potential harm caused by screening when the disease cannot be treated.

2. Test

It seems obvious to state, but the screening test itself must be appropriate. By this I mean that the test should be simple to administer and safe to use and should provide precise and validated results. It must also be acceptable for use with the target population. If a test for babies required anything more than them simply being in the room, most newborn screening tests would never get done. Beyond the ease and reliability of the test itself, if we are going to conduct a test, then we must decide what the results of the test mean. Think about tests you've taken in school. Let's say the pass mark is agreed to be 50%. Anything above 50% means you have passed; anything below means you fail the test. Screening tests are no different. Test values must be defined and agreed to decide whether someone is screen positive or negative. There must also be an agreed policy on the further diagnostic investigation that will be carried out for those who test positive. The UK government also specifies that tests focused on genetic variants and mutations must be kept under review, as these variants can of course change over time.

Let's pause for a second and talk a bit more about the test criteria, as it is vital to the success of screening programmes. Tests are not perfect. They can be wrong. This is why the validity and reliability of tests are so important. People will make decisions about their lives based on the results of screening tests, so the stakes are high. There are two possible errors that can occur. A false positive occurs when someone who does not in fact have the risk factors or early stages of a disease tests 'positive' due to error or statistical possibility. A false negative occurs when someone who does have the risk factors or early stages of the disease tests 'negative' despite actually having the disease. Both errors can cause harm: the former can cause unnecessary stress and further diagnostic tests; the latter can falsely reassure someone that nothing is wrong, when they are in fact ill. Thus, validity is crucial to screening.

The features of test validity
When considering how valid a test is, it is important to consider the following factors: Sensitivity, Specificity, Positive Predictive Value and Negative Predictive Value (Ruf et al., 2008 [2017]). What follows might seem a bit maths-y, but the ability of a test to show you whether someone needs further tests or treatment is crucial to being

able to deliver good population-level healthcare. Increasingly, there are tests for every-thing these days, but also big question marks over whether these tests are quality tests. By understanding a bit more about test validity—what it means and how to calculate it—as a healthcare professional, you're giving yourself the information you need to make important decisions about supporting your patients.

Sensitivity

The sensitivity of the test is the proportion of the people **with** the disease who **also** test positive—that is the detection rate of the test. Consider Figure 5.3. All these peo-ple have the disease. The test picks up 8 out of 10 people with the disease, therefore sensitivity is 80%. Not bad. A high sensitivity means the test is good at picking up the disease in the tested population.

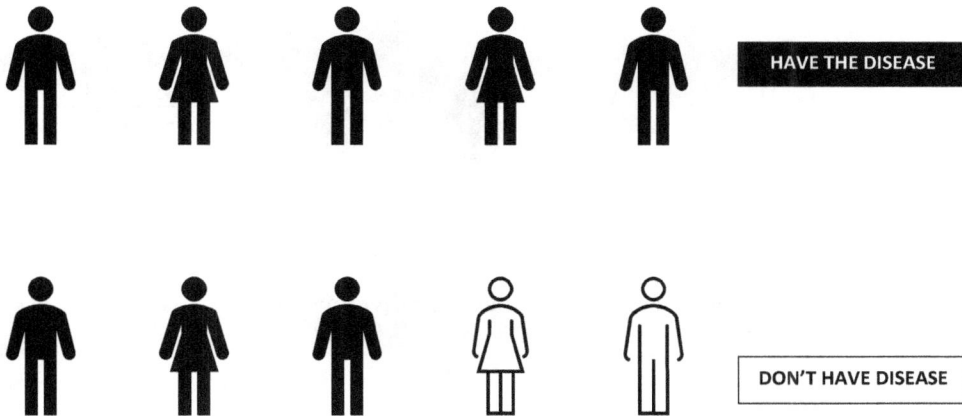

Figure 5.3 Sensitivity of a Screening Test.

The sensitivity of any given test is calculated by dividing true positives by true posi-tives + false negatives, using the following equation:

$$Sensitivity = \frac{a}{a+c}$$

Using Table 5.1, you can identify which values are a and c.

Table 5.1 Calculating the sensitivity of screening tests

Screening result	True state of patient		
	Disease present	Disease absent	Total
Positive test	a		
Negative test	c		
Total	a + c		

Specificity

Specificity is the proportion of people **without** the disease who **also** test negative—that is the detection rate of the test for those who DO NOT have the disease. In the example shown in Figure 5.4, none of these people have the disease. The test gives a negative result for 7 out of the 10 people who take it, giving a 70% specificity. High specificity means that a test is good at ruling out people who do not have the disease.

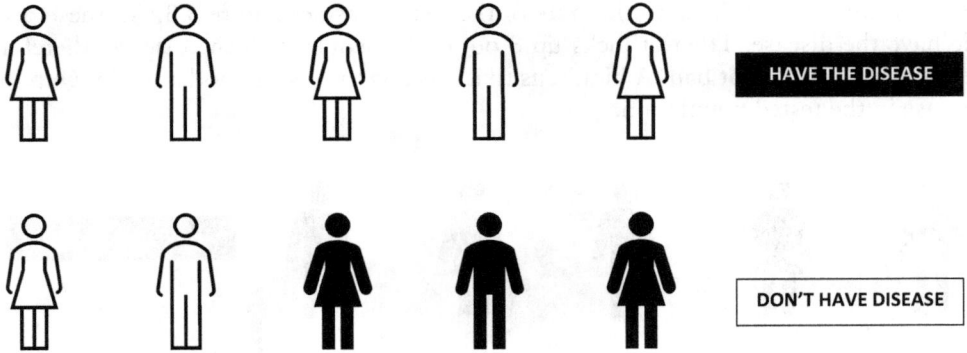

Figure 5.4 Specificity of a Screening Test.

The specificity of any given test is calculated by dividing true negatives by true negatives + false positives, using the equation below:

$$Specificity = \frac{d}{b+d}$$

Using Table 5.2, you can identify which values are b and d.

Table 5.2 Calculating the specificity of screening tests

Screening result	True state of patient		
	Disease present	Disease absent	Total
Positive test		b	
Negative test		d	
Total		b + d	

Sensitivity and specificity show the functionality of a test. When the same test is applied in the same way across populations, the test should always have the same sensitivity and specificity.

Positive Predictive Value (PPV)
Positive predictive value is the answer to the question:

If I test positive—what is my risk of actually having the disease?

The positive predictive value is the probability that someone who tests positive actually has the disease. This might seem an odd sentence to read, but remember that not all tests are 100% accurate, and many screening tests are not diagnostic tests for the disease. Instead, screening tests often identify markers that are known to be associated with a disease, but, on their own, are not enough to diagnose someone. Should someone test positive for these markers, further tests will help in making a diagnosis. PPV helps us to understand how good a test is at predicting the chance that someone has the disease.

The PPV of any given test is calculated by dividing true positives by true positives + false positives, using the equation below:

$$Specificity = \frac{a}{a+b}$$

Using Table 5.3, you can identify which values are a and b.

Table 5.3 Calculating the Positive Predictive Value of screening tests

Screening result	True state of patient		
	Disease present	Disease absent	Total
Positive test	a	b	a + b
Negative test			

Often, the more prevalent a disease in the population, the better the PPV. This is because there will be lots of true positives in the population for conditions that many people have, for example high blood pressure. Rare diseases have low prevalence, and so the PPV will not be as good, as the likelihood of the disease being present in the overall population is very low.

Negative Predictive Value (NPV)
Negative Predictive Value is the answer to the question:

If the screening test is negative—what are the chances that I genuinely don't have the disease?

This is the proportion of people who test negative and do not have the disease. It answers the question: out of all the people tested, how many of them genuinely do not have the disease?

The NPV of any given test is calculated by dividing true negatives by true negatives + false positives, using the equation below:

$$Specificity = \frac{d}{c+d}$$

Using Table 5.4, you can identify which values are c and d.

Table 5.4 Calculating the Negative Predictive Value of screening tests

Screening result	True state of patient		
	Disease present	Disease absent	Total
Positive test			
Negative test	c	d	c + d

3. Intervention

Once a valid test is identified, if you are going to screen for a disease, then there is an expectation that there will be effective intervention that patients can access, should the screening identify that they have the disease. This effective intervention must be evidence-based and there should be clear criteria and policies governing who is offered treatment and what the appropriate treatment is for that condition or disease. It could potentially be very harmful to screen a population for a disease or condition for which there are no available interventions or treatments. There should also be evidence that this intervention will lead to better outcomes when used in the pre- or early symptomatic stage. Otherwise, again, chances are that the screening programme will do more harm than good.

4. Screening programme

The screening programme has to be considered 'worth it'—not just in the way it improves overall population health but also in whether its costs are justified, both monetarily and with regards to potential harm to the people taking part. It needs to have a proven effectiveness in reducing mortality and morbidity, normally evidenced by high quality, randomised clinical trial data. In addition to being medically effective, it must also be a programme that is clinically, socially and ethically acceptable to doctors and the general public. So, for example: no forced screening of diseases or secret screening of diseases. Screening that required the loss of a limb would be unlikely to be allowed. In relation to this, the programme should be able to show that the benefits of being screened outweigh any harm from, for example overdiagnosis, overtreatment, false positives and inconclusive findings. Its cost must be balanced and proportionate to medical care more widely—basically, it should not cause harm and should be good value for money.

5. Implementation

Finally, before putting the screening programme into action, it must be ensured that all possible patient outcomes have been and can be optimised. This includes ensuring that all other options for managing the disease in question have been considered and discarded for good reason. There must be some form of quality assurance in place, which, importantly, means enough staff and facilities to run the programme effectively. There should also be high quality, but accessible, information available to the public; informed choice and informed consent must be ensured for potential and actual participants. The provided information should include scientific and clinical justifications for why the screening programme should exist, why it should be funded and why people should take part in it.

Is screening always the best option? And how do we know if it is even working?

As a result of the criteria above, we routinely evaluate our screening programmes. Screening programmes must be based on good quality evidence, but there is often public pressure to screen for conditions where screening may not be effective. A good example is prostate cancer. Despite being the most common cancer among men (1 in 8 men will have prostate cancer in their lifetimes), there is currently no screening programme for prostate cancer in the United Kingdom (Harris, 2023). When we consider the criteria above, it helps us understand why. Chiefly, there are issues with the second criterion: the test. The only existing test that can be used to screen prostate cancer, the prostate specific antigen (PSA) blood test, lacks validity (Harris, 2023). It does not accurately predict prostate cancer, and PSA levels can also be raised when no disease is present. As a result, a screening programme based on PSA blood tests would lead to some prostate cancer cases being missed, potential misdiagnoses in other cases and likely harm from unnecessary further interventions.

All of the above is before we even begin to unpack the more general difficulties with evaluating screening programmes (Kufe et al., 2003).

Evaluation difficulty #1: lead time bias

Lead time bias occurs when a screening programme appears to prolong survival, but in fact this is only because the screening programme allows for earlier diagnosis. Screened patients appear to survive longer, but only because they are diagnosed earlier. This is a 'false' increase: patients live for the same length of time regardless of when they are diagnosed, but with the screening programme, they spend longer knowing they have the disease. Figure 5.5 helps to explain how this works. In both cases, the person lives for the same amount of time, but screening allows for earlier diagnosis. When not properly understood, lead time bias can make it appear that screening programmes save more lives than they do.

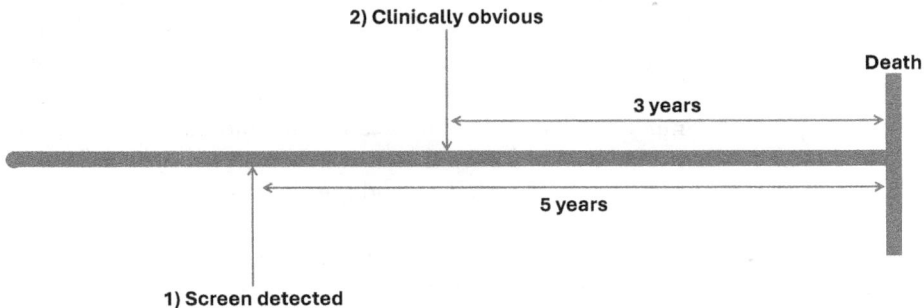

Figure 5.5 How Lead Time Bias Works.

Evaluation difficulty #2: length time bias

Screening programmes are often better at picking up slow-growing, unthreatening cases of disease such as cancer compared to aggressive, fast-growing ones (Kufe et al., 2003). This leads to a bias in the detection of less severe or threatening cancers in screening programmes. Diseases that are detectable through screening programmes are also more likely to have a favourable prognosis and, due to the inherent inaccuracy of screening, may have never led to a clinical issue at all.

Now, this is not as black and white as I am presenting here. Many of the diseases that we screen will cause problems and even death if they are not picked up. However, one serious criticism lobbied at screening programmes is that they, for the most part, are not looking for aggressive, acute diseases. Instead, they tend to go for the slow and steady silent growers. This leads to length time bias, resulting in a false conclusion that screening is lengthening lives when in fact those lives may not have been shortened by a later diagnosis because the disease itself is not very aggressive or life-limiting.

Evaluation difficulty #3: selection bias

Studies of screening are often skewed by what we can call the 'healthy volunteer' effect. People who engage in regular screening are also more likely to be engaging in other activities that protect them from disease. Think back to our discussion of health inequalities and inequities, and the kinds of people who present themselves for screening. Many people are eligible for screening but will never take part, for a variety of reasons that are not related to their health. Often, those who are already healthy—and have a long-term approach to remaining healthy over their lifetime—are more likely to take part in screening programmes. They are also more likely to be 'baseline' healthy to begin with. The result is selection bias in screening programmes, as the sample is not actually representative of the wider population.

The dark side of public health programmes: who is at fault for 'poor' health?

For the most part, public health programmes are trying to do a good thing—improve the health of a population in some way. However, when we take a wider, population-level view of health, these programmes have negative consequences at both the individual and population level. Take health promotion, for example. It might be hard to see how providing information about health behaviours and signs and symptoms of disease could cause harm, but it does.

Health promotion, though targeted at the population, often focuses on individual behavioural change. This means that the structural and socio-economic conditions that influence health are often not factored in (Bunton et al., 1995). Instead, health promotion downplays the impact of the wider socio-economic and environmental determinants of health, when we already know that these factors strongly influence the perceptions that individuals have of their health and the choices they make about their health.

This leads to a 'fallacy' of empowerment in health promotion. Giving people generic information about health does not automatically give them the power they need to make healthier choices. This leads to stigmatisation of people who do not appear to be engaging in healthy lifestyles. As we know from previous chapters, 'unhealthy' lifestyles are almost never due to ignorance or apathy. They are a result of adverse circumstances and wider socio-economic determinants of health throwing up barriers to good health.

I used to teach sociology of health in a medical school in the north of the United Kingdom. It was an incredibly deprived area. One of the things that we did there was ask the medical students to collect information on breastfeeding rates across the area for babies born in that year. In addition to high levels of deprivation, the area had low levels of breastfeeding mothers. Why do you think that is?

Ignorance on the importance of breastfeeding? Unlikely.

Wilfully ignoring the doctors' advice? Nope.

One of the main reasons is: nobody can stock shelves, clean houses or work the tills and breastfeed at the same time. Most people only get six weeks of maternity leave pay at 90% full pay and then Statutory Maternity Pay (SMP) for the next 33 weeks. By definition, SMP is considerably lower than most people's weekly take-home pay. In 2025, it is £184.03 per week or 90% of the person's average weekly earnings, whichever amount is lower (UK Government, n.d.b).

To give you some context, if someone is working 40 hours a week, that's an hourly wage of £4.60, and they're taxed on it too. Minimum wage in 2025 in the United Kingdom is at least £488.40 a week. This means that being on maternity leave, for most people, requires them to take a 63% pay cut. I don't know about you, but I couldn't survive on that. Many mothers simply cannot afford to go beyond that initial six-week period without getting into financial difficulty. And before you shove a breast pump at me—pumping at work is no picnic, believe me. Health promotion campaigns aimed at telling women that 'breast is best for the baby' create shame and stigma when mothers cannot act on that information. Instead of reframing breastfeeding as an option, we continue to see messages and policy aimed at mothers who engage in 'risky' bottle-feeding, when bottle-feeding is the only option they have. This is one of the big problems with health promotion—often there is no bridge between 'knowing why' and 'being able', but people still get judged all the same because they cannot cross the gulf between the two.

Screening programmes are not necessarily ethical either. To start with, there are serious and real concerns about whether the health service has the right to survey individual health (Bunton et al., 1995). What is done with the information regarding the results? Who owns that data? These are real questions that should be asked. The United Kingdom does not have an unblemished track record in managing screening programmes. In March 2025, it emerged that due to failures to invite eligible people to undergo screening programmes, at least ten people had died of a cancer for which they should have been screened (Gregory, 2025). This was not the first time this had happened; cases of screening programmes failing to invite the right people to take part have been reported again and again throughout the history of screening in the United Kingdom.

Finally, what about artificial intelligence (AI)? Increasingly, AI is seen as the way forward for screening, as it is thought to provide more efficient and cheaper ways of screening data such as CT and MRI scans. The NHS is currently trialling an AI programme called MIA to act as a second reader of mammogram scans (NHS England, 2025). Mammograms are normally read by two radiologists, independent of each other, to agree whether the mammogram shows areas of concern. MIA is being used as the 'second' reader, replacing the second radiographer by giving its opinion on the result of the mammogram (NHS England, 2025). The argument is that this frees up a radiographer to do other things, including more mammograms. However, AI is largely a black box in health. Most companies who design AI are not willing to share the details of their software, nor are they interested in taking on any liability should their product go wrong (NHS England, 2023). The result is that healthcare workers are increasingly being asked to use tools where no one will tell them how the tools are made or work, and neither will the toolmaker take responsibility should an error occur because of the tool. Thinking back to the features of test validity we discussed above, it is unclear whether AI successfully meets all those criteria; with the opaqueness of how AI works, it would also be difficult to independently determine its validity to the satisfaction of the standards to which we currently hold screening tests.

Conclusion

The promotion of health and wellbeing is, of course, a cornerstone of healthcare. This can be achieved at the individual level, where health and wellbeing can be improved using different tools to promote adherence to treatments. It can also be achieved at the population level, where public health programmes such as health promotion and screening work to improve awareness of disease and detection of disease. That being said, there remains much to be discovered and addressed in public health programmes. Whether they are wholly without harm remains an open question; historically, some have indeed caused harm, so the question does need to be asked and answered. The future is just as confusing. With AI already being used in breast screening, despite concerns around accuracy and accountability, it seems that the future of promoting health and wellbeing is likely to change rapidly in the next decade.

Test Yourself

1. Define 'concordance'.
2. What are the two key components of reflective listening?
   (a) Talking and Listening
   (b) Interrupting and Nodding
   (c) Mirroring and Paraphrasing
   (d) Understanding and Empathy
3. What is the focus of population and public health?
4. What are the four levels of prevention?
5. Health Promotion aims to:
   (a) Cure a disease once it has reached an advanced stage
   (b) Raise education and awareness about health, disease and illness
   (c) Detect and treat disease or risk factors at an early stage
   (d) Detect who needs palliative care

Note

1 If you are unfamiliar with Tuskegee, let me tell you about a truly dark time in recent medical history. The Tuskegee syphilis experiment, which started in 1932, was a programme of research where predominantly white scientists studied a group of Black men infected with syphilis in order to understand the full lifecycle of the disease. The men were told that they were being studied in order to investigate the effects of bad blood, and no informed consent was taken. This was initially conceived as a project to help justify better healthcare for these men; however, when it was discovered that penicillin could successfully treat syphilis, the participants were kept from and even denied access to penicillin so as to ensure that the data would be 'complete'—that is to ensure they died from the syphilis.

References

Adlife (n.d.). *University Hospitals Coventry & Warwickshire NHS trust*. Available at: https://adlifeproject.com/uhcw-nhs-trust

Arnold, S. and Jefferies, D. (2025). 'The NHS budget and how it has changed.' *The King's Fund*, 19th June. Available at: https://www.kingsfund.org.uk/insight-and-analysis/data-and-charts/nhs-budget-nutshell

Aronson, J.K. (2007). 'Compliance, concordance, adherence.' *British Journal of Clinical Pharmacology* 63(4): 383–384. https://doi.org/10.1111/j.1365-2125.2007.02893.x

Bank of England (2025). *Inflation calculator*. Available at: https://www.bankofengland.co.uk/monetary-policy/inflation/inflation-calculator [accessed 17th March 2025].

Benoit, C., Jeffery, A., Cleary, S., Masood, A., Paton, A. and Burt, C. (2023). *Health inequalities in Birmingham: Barriers encountered in underserved wards in East and West Birmingham*. Available at: https://research.aston.ac.uk/en/publications/health-inequalities-in-birmingham-barriers-encountered-in-underse

Buffington, A., Wenner, P., Brandenburg, D., Berge, J., Sherman, M. and Danner, C. (2016). 'The art of listening.' *Minnesota Medicine* 99(6): 46–48. Available at: https://www.adventhealth.com/sites/default/files/assets/buffington-a-the-art-of-listening.pdf

Bunton, R., Nettleton, S. and Burrows, R. (eds.) (1995). *The sociology of health promotion: critical analyses of consumption, lifestyle and risk*. London: Routledge.

Cochrane, A.L. and Holland, W.W. (1971). 'Validation of screening procedures.' *British Medical Bulletin* 27: 3–8. https://doi.org/10.1093/oxfordjournals.bmb.a070810

Department of Health and Social Care (2013). *'Catch it. Bin it. Kill it.' campaign to help reduce flu infections*. Available at: https://www.gov.uk/government/news/catch-it-bin-it-kill-it-campaign-to-help-reduce-flu-infections [accessed 21st May 2025].

Department of Health and Social Care (2018). *Prevention is better than cure*. Available at: https://assets.publishing.service.gov.uk/government/uploads/system/uploads/attachment_data/file/753688/Prevention_is_better_than_cure_5–11.pdf

Ewles, L. and Simnett, I. (2003). *Promoting health: A practical guide*. London: Bailhere Tindall Elsevier Limited.

Faculty of Public Health (2025). *Key areas of work in public health*. Available at: https://www.fph.org.uk/what-is-public-health/key-areas-of-work-in-public-health/ [accessed 1st April 2025].

Gregory, A. (2025). 'Ten died of cancer after NHS blunder in England meant they were not invited for screening.' *The Guardian*, 11th March. Available at: https://www.theguardian.com/society/2025/mar/11/ten-died-of-cancer-after-nhs-england-blunder-meant-they-were-not-invited-for-screening

Harris, M. (2023). 'UK NSC welcomes major new prostate cancer screening research.' *UK National Screening Committee*, 20th November. Available at: https://nationalscreening.blog.gov.uk/2023/11/20/uk-nsc-welcomes-major-new-prostate-cancer-screening-research/

HM Treasury (2018). *Soft drinks industry levy comes into effect*. Available at: https://www.gov.uk/government/news/soft-drinks-industry-levy-comes-into-effect [accessed 2nd April 2025].

Kim, J., Combs, K., Downs, J. and Tillman, F., III. (2018). 'Medication adherence: The elephant in the room.' *U.S. Pharmacist* 43: 30–34. Available at: https://www.uspharmacist.com/article/medication-adherence-the-elephant-in-the-room

Kisling, L.A. and Das, J.M. (2023). *Prevention strategies*. StatPearls Publishing. Available at: https://www.ncbi.nlm.nih.gov/books/NBK537222/

Kottke, T.E., Faith, D.A., Jordan, C.O., Pronk, N.P, Thomas, R.J. and Capewell, S. (2009). 'The comparative effectiveness of heart disease prevention and treatment strategies.' *American Journal of Preventive Medicine* 36(1): 82–88. https://doi.org/10.1016/j.amepre.2008.09.010

Kufe, D.W., Pollock, R.E., Weichselbaum, R.R., Bast, R.C., Jr., Gansler, T.S., Holland, J.F. and Frei, E., III. (eds.) (2003). *Cancer medicine*. Hamilton, ON: BC Decker.

McVean, A. (2019). '40 years of human experimentation in America: The Tuskegee study.' *Office for Science and Society*, 25th January. Available at: https://www.mcgill.ca/oss/article/history/40-years-human-experimentation-america-tuskegee-study [accessed 21st May 2025].

NHS England (2023). *Liability*. Available at: https://digital-transformation.hee.nhs.uk/building-a-digital-workforce/dart-ed/horizon-scanning/understanding-healthcare-workers-confidence-in-ai/chapter-3-governance/liability

NHS England (2025). *Understand AI*. Available at: https://transform.england.nhs.uk/ai-lab/explore-all-resources/understand-ai/

Paton, A. (2019). '"Being Guided": What oncofertility patients' decisions can teach us about the efficacy of autonomy, agency and decision-making theory in the contemporary clinical encounter.' *International Journal of Feminist Approaches to Bioethics* 12(2): 18–35. https://doi.org/10.3138/ijfab.12.2.02

Ruf, M., Morgan, O. and Mackenzie, K. (2008 [2017]). 'Statistical aspects of screening tests, including knowledge of and ability to calculate, sensitivity, specificity, positive and negative predictive values, and the use of ROC curves.' *Health Knowledge*. Faculty of Public Health. Available at: https://www.healthknowledge.org.uk/public-health-textbook/disease-causation-diagnostic/2c-diagnosis-screening/statistical-aspects-screening

Sabaté, E. (2003). *Adherence to long term therapies: Evidence for action*. Geneva: World Health Organization. Available at: https://iris.who.int/bitstream/handle/10665/42682/9241545992.pdf [accessed 17th March 2025].

Scales, R., Miller, J. and Burden, R. (2003). 'Why wrestle when you can dance? Optimizing outcomes with motivational interviewing.' *Journal of the American Pharmacists Association* 43(5 Suppl 1): S46–7. https://doi.org/10.1331/154434503322612456

Stein, R.F. and Hurd, S.N. (eds.) (2000). *Using student teams in the classroom: A faculty guide*. Anker Publishing Company.

Street, R.L., Jr., Makoul, G., Arora, N.K. and Epstein, R.M. (2009). 'How does communication heal? Pathways linking clinician-patient communication to health outcomes.' *Patient Education and Counseling* 74: 295–301. https://doi.org/10.1016/j.pec.2008.11.015

Stubbe, D.E. (2018). 'The therapeutic alliance: The fundamental element of psychotherapy.' *Focus* 16(4): 402–403. https://doi.org/10.1176/appi.focus.20180022

Thomas, T. (2024). 'UK sugar tax explained: What is it and has it worked?' *The Guardian*, 9th July. Available at: https://www.theguardian.com/business/article/2024/jul/09/uk-sugar-tax-explained-what-is-it-and-has-it-worked [accessed 2nd April 2025].

UK Government (n.d.a). *Population screening programmes*. Available at: https://www.gov.uk/health-and-social-care/population-screening-programmes [accessed 2nd April 2025].

UK Government (n.d.b). *Maternity pay and leave*. Available at: https://www.gov.uk/maternity-pay-leave/pay

UK National Screening Committee (2022). *Criteria for a population screening programme*. Available at: https://www.gov.uk/government/publications/evidence-review-criteria-national-screening-programmes/criteria-for-appraising-the-viability-effectiveness-and-appropriateness-of-a-screening-programme [accessed 2nd April 2025].

UK National Screening Committee (2025). *2021 to 2022 data from England underlines huge impact of national NHS screening programmes*. Available at: https://nationalscreening.

blog.gov.uk/2025/01/30/2021-to-2022-data-from-england-underlines-huge-impact-of-national-nhs-screening-programmes/#:~:text=an%20estimated%204%2C500%20lives%20being,every%20year%20in%20the%20UK [accessed 21st May 2025].

Usherwood, T. (2017). 'Encouraging adherence to long-term medication.' *Australian Prescriber* 40(4): 147–150. https://doi.org/10.18773/austprescr.2017.050

van Dulmen, S., Sluijs, E., van Dijk, L., de Ridder, D., Heerdink, R. and Bensing, J. (2007). 'Patient adherence to medical treatment: A review of reviews.' *BMC Health Services Research* 7: 55. https://doi.org/10.1186/1472-6963-7-55

Wilson, J.M.G. and Jungner, G. (1968). *Principles and practice of screening for disease.* World Health Organisation. Available at: https://iris.who.int/handle/10665/37650

World Health Organisation (1986). *Ottawa charter for health promotion.* Available at: https://www.who.int/healthpromotion/conferences/previous/ottawa/en/index3.html

York Health Economics Consortium (2010). *Evaluation of the scale, causes and costs of waste medicines.* Available at: https://discovery.ucl.ac.uk/id/eprint/1350234/1/Evaluation_of_NHS_Medicines_Waste__web_publication_version.pdf

Zeitouny, S., Cheng, L., Wong, S.T., Tadrous, M., McGrail, K. and Law, M.R. (2023). 'Prevalence and predictors of primary nonadherence to medications prescribed in primary care.' *Canadian Medical Association Journal* 195(30): E1000–E1009. https://doi.org/10.1503/cmaj.221018

CHAPTER 6

Politics and health

Politics and health are entangled in a way that can never be unravelled. As we saw earlier, political decisions, and the political ideologies that inform these decisions, strongly impact on health, even when those decisions, policies and practices are not explicitly about health itself. Political ideology is as important to good health as diet, exercise and genetics. Indeed, hopefully by now it has become clear just how much outside forces such as politics and policy can change the health of an individual, community or population for the worse.

The best way to understand the impact that politics has on health is through a case study. In this book we will use the United Kingdom and the National Health Service (NHS). We will start right at the beginning, showing how political ideology shaped and gave birth to the NHS. We will move through time to the important two decades between 2000 and 2020 that are reshaping healthcare now, then finally end with a more practical discussion of the way politics will impact your daily practice through rationing and resource allocation.

In the beginning

The NHS was established on 5th July 1948. Its origin story has long passed into lore. It is the story of a great man, Beveridge, who saw a new way of supporting society, and of Bevan, the architect who made that vision a reality by creating the NHS. However, while the United Kingdom was the first European country to offer free healthcare at the point of access, the NHS was, and is, much more about political ideology than anything else (Klein, 2006, p. 1). In fact, the roots of the NHS can be seen more than 30 years before 1948, during the two world wars. The economic depression and resulting deprivation in the interwar years brought to light the sorry state of health in which many lived (Clement, 2023).

While the Second World War was far from won, the coalition government of the time began surveying the health and social care landscape of Britain in 1941. A year later,

DOI: 10.4324/9781032677552-6

the damning Beveridge Report identified what Beveridge theatrically (but with reason) called 'The Five Giants' that were afflicting Britain: Want, Disease, Ignorance, Squalor and Idleness (Beveridge, 1942). As with many political decisions, while tackling these giants (or 'Evils' as they were also called, which shows how these concepts were viewed politically) was likely the right thing to do, it was the political and economic argument that really helped sell a better health and social care system. Beveridge and his allies argued that only by creating a system that would combat these 'evils' could the United Kingdom recover from the war years and succeed economically, socially and politically (Clement, 2023). Better still, doing so would likely be affordable (Harris, 1977, p. 412). A political win-win.

Though people did have to pay to read it (about £4 in 2025 money), the Beveridge Report captured the popular, political and social imagination of the period and was seen as a blueprint for a comprehensive welfare state (Clement, 2023). With Beveridge, the political concept of the 'state' caring for citizens from the cradle to the grave was born, and thus, for the first time in several centuries, good health was not solely viewed as a personal responsibility. Note my word choice above: the political concept of state healthcare. That is deliberate. The way a healthcare system is designed, funded and supported is a political decision, made by a governing power and based on a political ideology. While health may be viewed by some as a good within itself, politics certainly does not see it that way. Recall, in the introduction, our discussion of the different ways people understand and view health. These beliefs bleed into governments, influencing the decisions they make and the policies they create.

State-run healthcare was so strong a political concept that both the Conservative and Labour parties campaigned on it, and Labour's 1945 victory was strongly enabled by their promise to develop a welfare state with all the necessary services laid out in the Beveridge Report: what Hennessy so wonderfully calls offering the public the 'Full Beveridge' (Hennessy, 2022). It should be noted that the idea of state-run healthcare was pushing against a door that had been slowly opening more and more since the early 1900s. There was a wider, post-war political view that the rubble of the last 30 years should give rise to something new (Day, 2017). Political rhetoric at the time dismissed the idea of patching a broken system, and the NHS was the shiny example of this will to improve by making something wholly new (UK Government, 1945). The period was also marked by a political push to nationalise services more generally, for which health and social care were a natural fit (Hansard, 1945).

Despite this, the road to the welfare state in Britain was bumpy. The Beveridge Report's findings took the then government by surprise in terms of the scale of the solution recommended. Like any political issue, of which, again, healthcare is one, there were various political concerns about the 'optics' of a welfare system in the United Kingdom. Both the Chancellor, Kingsley Wood, and Churchill's advisor, Lord Cherwell, expressed reservations to the Prime Minister about a proposed system that would see, for example, a pauper and a millionaire receive the same pension (Day, 2017). In addition, Beveridge was suggesting the implementation of a system far superior to the health and social care system in the United States, which, incidentally, was effectively bankrolling the United Kingdom's recovery from the war (Day, 2017). Not necessarily a good look, politically. For a brief moment, the NHS almost never was, simply to spare Britain and America's political blushes.

A political hot potato if there ever was one. And what does the political world do with a hot potato? They either cover it up or leak it. Leaking it is precisely what Beveridge's allies are alleged to have done in order to ensure the report's publication, with the Minister of Information, Brendan Brachen, telling Churchill that 'Beveridge's friends are playing politics [. . .] and when the report arrives there will be an immense ballyhoo about the importance of implementing the recommendations without delay' (Day, 2017).

Can you really blame people for making a 'ballyhoo' about better healthcare, better housing, better national insurance and better support in unemployment? Britain's population at the time was often jobless, living in slums, squalor or rubble with no health benefits. Of course there was a societal need for a welfare state and of course the public wanted it. The government knew it too but were panicked by the cost and scale of delivering one.

Additionally, and perhaps surprisingly to the modern healthcare professional, doctors weren't keen on a nationalised health service either. The British Medical Association (BMA), amongst other medical professional bodies, were none too happy with nationalising health, and GPs in particular voted overwhelmingly against the idea (Lambert, 2024). Before you get angry, remember a couple of important things. First, universal state-funded healthcare was unheard of in Europe or North America, so the western health tradition had no real experience of what it would look like or mean for healthcare professionals. Next, don't forget that the BMA is a trade union. It's their job to protect the jobs of doctors. A new way of organising and funding healthcare was a threat to those jobs. Finally, they weren't the only ones. The American Medical Association (AMA) launched a vicious campaign against state-run and funded healthcare in 1949 in response to Truman's election. It remains one of the most steadfast political and public relations attacks in the western medicine tradition. Recently, research has shown that the impact and influence of the AMA's attack, which likened nationalised healthcare to socialism, is likely one of the key reasons why the United States remains a fee-for-service system (Alsan et al., 2024; Marks, 2022). This is another example of how deeply political ideology influences health and healthcare provision.

While this opposition from doctors led to very different healthcare systems, it still has a legacy within the NHS—though, granted, not as strong as in the United States. The political negotiations needed to get the doctors onside for the NHS means that the service has never been the monolith that so many of us perceive. Instead, it is a patchwork of services, delivered by different providers, across different systems throughout the devolved nations. If that sounds like a hot mess, it's because sometimes it is. I would like to skip ahead now to dive into the way the NHS works in the present day and the political influences on those inner workings.

And then there was devolution: how the healthcare system in the United Kingdom works

The most crucial aspect of the relationship between health and politics, in terms of individual and population health, is the way the healthcare system works. What this system is, what its various parts are, how it is deployed in a country, how its citizens access it (or don't) is a really important part of health. It is worth taking a quick detour to look at the four main ways healthcare systems work across the world, before settling in to learn about how the NHS itself works, as these concepts are largely politically driven.

The four basic models of healthcare provision

Out of pocket model

Most countries in the world do not have universal healthcare provision for their citizens or free healthcare at the point of access (Reid, 2010). In those countries, only people who are rich enough receive healthcare; others do not. It is genuinely that simple. Some have public hospitals that provide free emergency care, but only emergency care. Thereafter, all costs are borne by the patient. Those who can afford to do so pay for healthcare insurance so that they do not have to pay all the expenses associated with their healthcare. Many people believe this is the American model, but that's not quite accurate. It is the case for about 8% of Americans that they have absolutely no insurance or support to pay for healthcare (Keisler-Starkey and Bunch, 2024), but other countries have much higher rates, for example Cambodia, where about 60% of the population have to pay out of pocket for healthcare (Kaiser et al., 2025). Sometimes also referred to as the Individual Liability model, this model is associated with the political ideas that underpin libertarianism. Libertarianism is a good example of the strong link between politics and health, as it is the bedrock of many health-care systems worldwide and thus influences hundreds of millions of health outcomes every year. Libertarianism prioritises individual autonomy and freedom—people are responsible for themselves and no one else. Libertarians are not huge fans of state power or, often, state health, viewing public health (and all public services) as interference from the 'nanny state' (BBC, 2024). I would love to know how many libertarians remain steadfast to this ideology after they have to pay off an enormous healthcare bill. If you are looking for a research project, might I humbly suggest that one. Inquiring minds want to know.

Bismarck model

This model is named after Otto von Bismarck, Chancellor of Prussia, who created a welfare state in 1883 as part of the unification of Germany. Under the Bismarck model, healthcare is delivered by private healthcare providers financed by an insurance system. Normally not-for-profit 'sickness funds' are strictly regulated and jointly funded by employers and employees through payroll deduction. It is a multi-payer insurance model that uses multiple sources of funding to provide healthcare; in most countries where it is used, it also provides universal healthcare access, regardless of wealth. Examples include Germany, France, Belgium, Netherlands, Switzerland, and Japan.

The Bismarck model has an odd political legacy. On the one hand, it is a shining example of what is required when a state adopts a policy of social support for its citizens. On the other, like so many great things in health, it could have been a political accident. As we saw with the creation of the NHS, the Bismarck model was as much a strategy to get one over on political opponents as it was to create universal health coverage. One historian suggests that Bismarck himself didn't even care much what it was called or what it did, as long as the population knew that it was HIS government that had instituted healthcare reform, not his opposition, the Social Democrats (Boissoneault, 2017). A global healthcare revolution borne of extreme political pettiness. Love it.

The National Health Insurance model

Likely named after Lloyd George's National Insurance Act (1911) in the United Kingdom, after which employers and employees began paying National Insurance contributions, it is actually Canada that is best known for using this model. Healthcare is delivered by private healthcare providers financed by a government-run insurance scheme funded by citizens' contributions. It is a single-payer scheme (the government), which gives little incentive for marketisation of healthcare, and provides strong bargaining and buying power to the government when they negotiate healthcare service rates. It is relatively cheap to run, as there is only one provider (unlike the complex multi-provider insurance systems in the United States), and is a not-for-profit system. In addition to Canada, examples include Taiwan and South Korea. The National Health Insurance model shares its roots with the NHS; it was born out of the growing political will during the first four decades of the twentieth century to improve support for the population through a welfare state that delivered necessary public services, such as healthcare, to improve people's overall lives.

The Beveridge model

The Beveridge model is a version of the National Health Insurance model with a small but significant change: it is a single-payer and single-provider model, meaning that the government both pays for and delivers the healthcare. Healthcare is universally available to all citizens, for free, at the point of access. It is delivered mostly by state-controlled healthcare providers and financed by the government through general taxation. Examples include the United Kingdom, Spain, most Scandinavian countries, New Zealand and Cuba. As we saw earlier in the chapter, and above in the National Health Insurance model, the Beveridge model grew from the political belief that the state has a responsibility towards the health and wellbeing of is citizens and must provide services to support that health and wellbeing.

Healthcare in the United Kingdom

While the NHS is held up as 'the' model of universal healthcare, it is not just one entity, but instead a many-headed beast that serves several different functions. So how does it work? First, you have to remember that the United Kingdom is made up of four nations: England, Wales, Scotland and Northern Ireland. Each has their own systems of government and public services that serve their respective populations. Money, via taxation, flows from the UK government to the treasury and is then disseminated across the four nations and whichever body manages their version of the NHS in their country. As a result, when you see, for example, the Chief Executive speaking about the NHS, they are actually speaking about NHS England. They do not speak for the Directorate for Health and Social Care in Scotland, nor do they speak for NHS Scotland. In fact, you may be surprised to learn that we do not have shared or standardised policies and practices in the NHS across the United Kingdom. Indeed, they are often different between nations, regions and even local trusts (Figure 6.1).

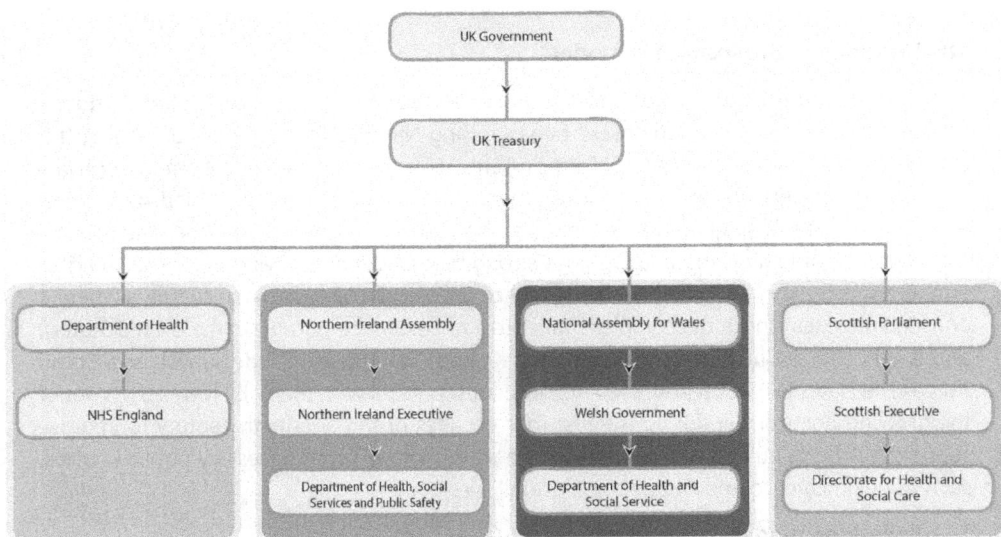

Figure 6.1 Funding of the Healthcare System in the United Kingdom. Due to announcements in March 2025, this is now slightly out-of-date, but no new system has been announced yet (Doheny, 2015).

Let's consider England first, as it is home to the Department of Health and Social Care, which has a wide range of responsibilities across healthcare in the United Kingdom, not just England. For example, the Medicines and Healthcare Products Regulatory Agency (MHRA) is the body that decides which medicines and medical technologies are safe to use in the United Kingdom. Then NICE decides the policies and procedures for using those medicines—where, when, for who and what dose.

Among other things, such as the Care Quality Commission, Health Education England and whatever the government in power calls the UK's public health service, until 2025 the Department of Health and Social Care provided funding to NHS England, which funded and ran the NHS in England. In 2023/2024 this amounted to a budget of £171 billion (Arnold and Jefferies, 2025). From there, money, policy and practice flowed into services such as GP practices, hospitals and, perhaps surprisingly, private practice (because private practice a) still receives money for carrying out services that the NHS does not/cannot and b) regardless of where its money comes from is still subject to the same best practice and policies as the NHS). The entirety of this process is regulated by the Care Quality Commission (the CQC).

In March 2025, the UK government announced they were abolishing NHS England, describing it as an unwieldy, inefficient and expensive administrative beast (Triggle and Catt, 2025). As of this writing (two months later), information has been thin on the ground about its replacement. During the last three years, the NHS in England has been restructured twice, largely to try and keep the ship afloat amidst rising costs, rising needs and a dwindling budget. It is interesting to note that a key part of the decision to abolish NHS England is political: the Prime Minister noted that NHS England was the 'world's largest quango', meaning a Quasi-Autonomous Non-Governmental Organisation (Triggle and Catt, 2025). Quangos are interesting political entities. They are funded by the taxpayer, but they are not controlled directly by central government. Other examples in the United Kingdom include Network Rail, the Environment Agency and the Gambling Commission (Triggle and Catt, 2025). It is true that, for years, people have felt that NHS England was becoming too bloated. It is also true that devolved control at the local level works very well for healthcare systems, as each locality will have slightly different funding needs. However, it cannot be ignored that this is still a political decision, not a clinical one, which will have significant consequences on how healthcare is delivered in England. As I sit in a Greene King pub (it was the only restaurant close by; don't give me a hard time!) in May 2025 writing this chapter and listening to news speculation on the future of the NHS, it remains to be seen whether those consequences will be positive or negative.

To try and understand how healthcare might be delivered in England moving forward, let's start by looking at what NHS England was until March 2025.

Since 2022, NHS England has been organised into Integrated Care Systems (ICSs), which are partnerships that bring together providers and commissioners of NHS services with local authorities and other local partners to plan, coordinate and commission health and care services within one geographic area. Previously in England there was an internal market approach to the way healthcare was delivered—meaning that competition for contracts from internal and external providers drove service provision. Trusts were also largely autonomous in the way they acted. In ICSs, the focus is on collaboration, with the aim of harmonising health and care organisations so that they can work together. The idea is that integrating health and care services will increase efficiency, improve the overall health service and as a result, improve population health. As you can see, the NHS in England tends to reinvent itself every couple of governments. Often, everything old is new again, but I hope this gives you a good idea of how the overall system works, regardless of what things are called or the exact specifics of how the money flows (Figure 6.2).

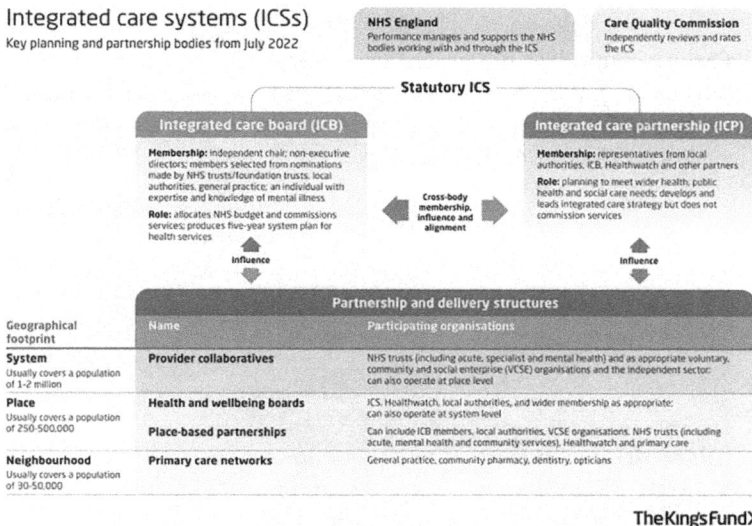

Figure 6.2 Integrated Care Systems in England. Please note that this image is out-of-date following the March 2025 announcement, but again, no new system has been proposed to replace it (The King's Fund, 2022).

Scotland also uses an integrated care approach to healthcare organisation (Scottish Government, n.d.). It has used this approach for longer than England, so by looking to Scotland it is possible to get a sense of where Integrated Care Systems could be in England in a few years' time. The focus in Scotland is on joining up services so that the organisations planning, buying and providing publicly-funded healthcare—including mental health, community care services and preventative health services—are available to the population of a geographical area based on their needs. As well as the NHS, the organisations include local authorities and independent care providers so that clinical services are aligned with social care services. You can see in Figure 6.3 that despite also being an integrated care model, Scotland is organised differently to England, in terms of not just what things are called but also where the money goes and the services included (Figure 6.3).

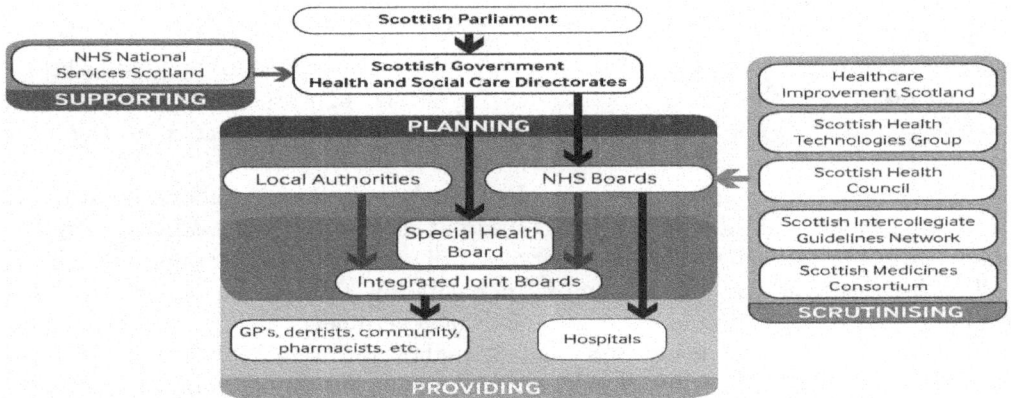

Figure 6.3 Integrated Care System in Scotland (Doheny, 2015).

Wales tells another familiar integrated care story, but spends a significant amount of time and money on public health and health prevention programmes. Again, just as Scotland is different to England, Wales spends more resources on preventative care than the other nations (Figure 6.4).

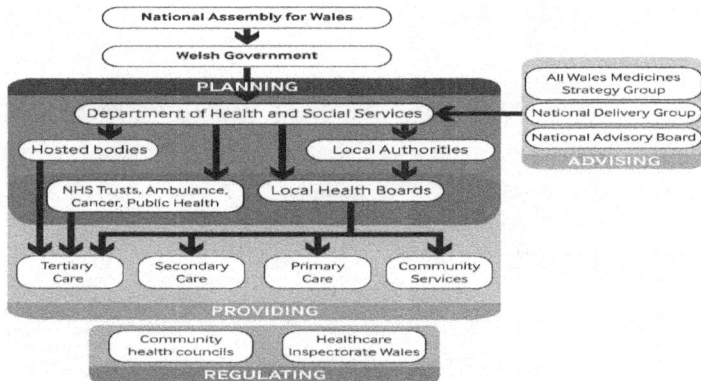

Figure 6.4 Integrated Care System in Wales (Doheny, 2015).

Finally, Northern Ireland also has a different way of governing itself and thus a different way of organising its healthcare. Northern Ireland has a Health and Social Care Service (HSC), sometimes called the NHS, but healthcare alone is not the only function of the HSC. Care in Northern Ireland is perhaps more integrated, as social services are part of the Health and Social Care Service. The social services are provided by local councils (Figure 6.5).

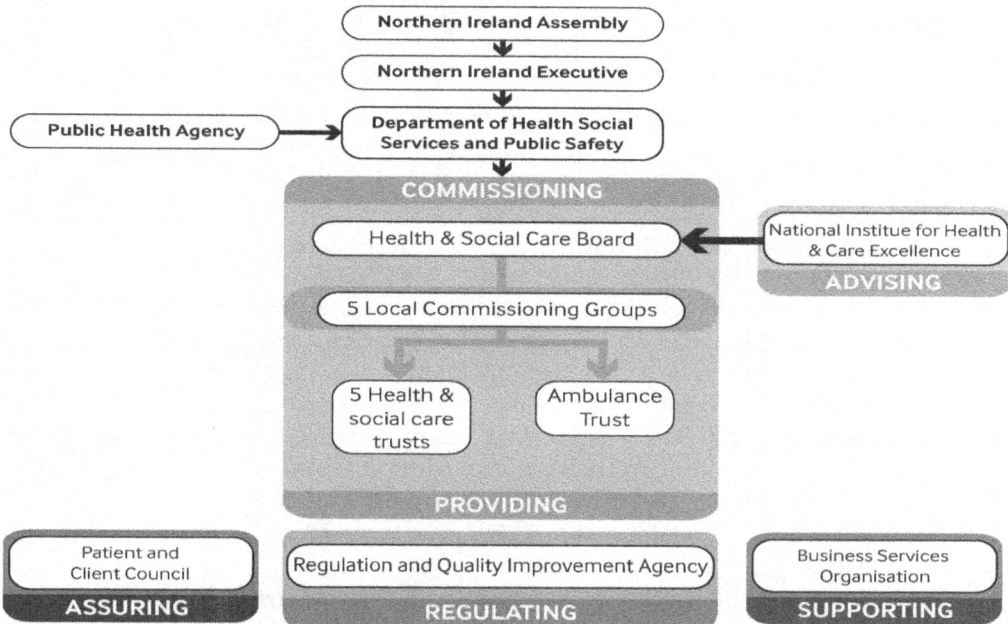

Figure 6.5 Northern Ireland's Health and Social Care Service (Doheny, 2015).

Confused? It's understandable.

So how do all these different healthcare systems, which are supposed to be in the same country, funded by the same government and governed by the same regulations, compare with each other? For the most part, it is the same provision of healthcare, but with tweaks to the way it is funded, accessed by patients and governed (Bevan et al., 2014). Each of these 'tweaks' are actually political decisions made by the government of that nation based on what it is willing to fund and supply to the population. For example, Scotland and Wales offer more services, such as free prescriptions (prescriptions are paid in England). Northern Ireland pools its health and social care budget, while the other three nations keep them largely separate. England has a quasi-market in healthcare that still uses private providers. The result of devolved healthcare is devolved health outcomes—by this I mean that people's life expectancy and overall health will differ depending on where they live and receive healthcare. For example, life expectancy is highest in England and lowest in Scotland (Office of National Statistics, 2024). This has little to do with deep fried Mars bars and a lot to do with the accessibility of healthcare in each region.

In the last of days: how politics destroyed healthcare in the United Kingdom in 20 short years

It is by looking at the two decades between 2000 and 2020 that it is possible to see just how influential politics is on health. The NHS of 2025 is the result of decisions made in government about what to prioritise and what to leave behind. During those 20 years, the NHS weathered political interest that at times improved it and at other times contributed to its current decline. These highs and lows were based on political decisions, not medical or clinical ones. They were political because they were also mostly financial decisions about the amount of money that the NHS should receive to deliver healthcare to the nation. Richard Murray, Chief Executive of the King's Fund, explains it well in his report on the NHS during those years: 'rather than attributing the current situation to some inevitable built-in decay, [the report] draws out the decisions (or lack of them) that have led to the current crisis' (Ham, 2023). In this, he is clear that the NHS didn't just decline. People, that is people in government, made decisions that *made* it decline.

At the dawn of the new millennium, the NHS wasn't doing so well. A particularly difficult winter in 1999/2000 had shown up an NHS in crisis (Ham, 2023). In response, the Labour government in power increased NHS funding so that it could provide better care through the NHS Plan (UK Government, 2000). It was an ambitious plan, not just limited to more staff or more pay; it also involved the creation of targets, development of performance management systems, inspections and regulation (Ham, 2023). The ambition of the Labour government paid off. During this period (around 2000–2008), wait times were at a minimum, halving across most areas of care (National Audit Office, 2010). Regulation, especially around resources, also played a key role in a more efficient NHS, as NICE, established in 1999, set clear guidelines on the use of drugs, interventions and treatments (NICE, 2024).

As the decade moved on, the NHS was seen to move from strength to strength; public satisfaction with the service grew with it, reaching its peak in 2010 (Wellings et al., 2022). You may be wondering why this chapter about politics and health seems to be about history instead, but the point is this: much like its inception in 1948, the NHS was thriving in the 2000s because there was a political will to improve, which meant the NHS was being prioritised by the government, which translated into more money for the NHS overall. How much exactly? Well, the previous Conservative government had spent just 2.8% of its overall budget on healthcare, while the Labour government of the early 2000s spent 5.6%, double that of its political predecessor (Arnold and Jefferies, 2025).

Then came 15th September 2008, and the world was plunged into a global financial crisis and recession. The financial priorities of governments everywhere shifted, including the United Kingdom. The country then had a new government. In the United Kingdom, 2010 saw a new, coalition government formed between the Conservatives and the Liberal Democrats. This partnership would set the NHS on a different path in the 2010s, one that set in motion more than a decade of decline in the service.

Almost immediately, the focus shifted to fiscal responsibility and reducing the deficit. Public services were frozen or cut, and soon the NHS was caught in the crosshairs of Chancellor George Osborne's 'austerity' decade (BBC News, 2011). In October 2010,

£81 billion of spending cuts were announced, in which the NHS was included; more importantly, related services such as social care, housing and education saw their budgets slashed (Ham, 2023). While the previous Labour government had spent 5.6% of the overall budget on health, the coalition years saw that drop to just 1% (Arnold and Jefferies, 2025). The result? Not only were healthcare services underfunded throughout the 2010s, with little investment in infrastructure, equipment and workforce, but services that cared for people outside the NHS no longer existed either (Ham, 2023). This meant that as the decade of austerity chugged on, there was less community care, less home help, less housing and less support in schools for those who needed it most. Unable to access services that used to exist, people now went into hospital instead, putting increased strain on a system that was already trying to do more with significantly less (Age UK, 2024).

By 2014/2015, NHS trusts were getting into financial difficulty and the NHS deficit started to grow (Appleby et al., 2015). Political decisions to promote competition and restructure the NHS further damaged the already fragile service (Ham, 2023). Despite several warnings, what followed, up until the COVID-19 pandemic of 2020, was a series of political promises that were never really fulfilled and a stalwart insistence from the government in power that they could not meet the financial needs of the NHS (Ham, 2023). While the Conservative majority government formed in 2015 invested more in the NHS, with around 2.3% of the overall budget spent on health, this was still only half of the funding that had seen the NHS thrive in previous decades. It should also be noted that some of this reported increase is misleading, as it can be attributed to increased spending during the pandemic (Arnold and Jefferies, 2025). The result is that in 2025, 25 years after a political commitment to improve the NHS, further financial and service cuts are on the horizon, as another new government tries to grapple with a decade and a half of neglect so they can balance the books (Triggle, 2025).

Of course, let us not forget that our healthcare is devolved, meaning not all decisions are taken in Westminster, but that doesn't stop the political bickering. The healthcare systems in Scotland and Wales, for example, have been shaped by their dominant parties over the years too, chiefly Labour and SNP, who have looked to differentiate themselves from Westminster—though to be fair, the extent to which they can successfully do this is constrained by the funding of devolution. Scotland and Wales blame Westminster for not being able to deliver the health services that are needed in their countries. The Conservatives blame the financial crises and economy for not allowing more money to flow from Westminster to the devolved health services when they were in power. Labour blames the Conservatives for the mess the NHS finds itself in now, regardless of which country it is in. And so on and so on. Meanwhile the NHS suffers a tragedy of the commons, with no one willing to take the responsibility, let alone the blame for the current state of affairs.

The above is really a series of political decisions that has led to an NHS that is unsafe in 2025 and unlikely to become safer unless political will sees fit to prioritise it once again—by which I mean provide the necessary funding to allow the NHS to work to its full potential (Paton, 2023). Until then, it is unlikely that there will be any positive change in the system and healthcare in the United Kingdom will continue to decline (Paton, 2022). It's a sorry state of affairs, and one that shows why understanding the politics behind healthcare is as important as understanding healthcare itself. It is also the reason why resource allocation and rationing are part of everyday medical life.

And Jesus wept: resource allocation, rationing and the way politics influences your daily clinical practice

So far, we have discussed in general terms how politics impact on health and healthcare, but this is not just an abstract influence or something you can ignore in your daily practice. In this section, I want to discuss how current politics and the growing, aging and ailing population will affect you day to day. Again, we will use the NHS as our case study. The NHS is, and has been, at crisis point for some time (Darzi, 2024). There are fewer and fewer resources—whether they be hospitals, beds or staff—available to care for patients. As outlined above, the current and past United Kingdom governments have not prioritised the NHS or the associated services that take strain off the NHS such as community and social services. For many of you reading this chapter, this environment of scarce resources and an NHS on its knees is going to be your working environment. An environment where you never have enough of what you need to do the best job you can. This is why I want to spend some time explaining resource allocation and rationing and how it is used in the healthcare system. You are going to need to understand why resources are rationed and allocated and how decisions are made about the services you can offer your patients. Why? Because at the end of the day, when you can't give your patient something because there isn't enough of it or it is too expensive for the NHS to cover, you are the one that delivers that bad news and you are the one that has to come up with an alternative solution. Forewarned is forearmed, and all that.

Before we begin, a quick word about terminology. 'Rationing' and 'healthcare' are not words that societies like to hear in the same sentence. In the United Kingdom, this has led to lots of euphemistic words to try and soften the fact that we use rationing ALL OF THE TIME in the NHS. This tends to send people into a panic, so instead we use friendly words like 'priority setting'. It sounds much nicer than 'we need to figure out how few things we can get away with giving patients because we are running out of the things/services/doctors etc.'. 'Priority setting' rolls off the tongue much more easily.

Priority setting 'describes decisions about the allocation of resources between the competing claims of different services, different patient groups or different elements of care' (Klein, 2010). This sounds okay, right? Not too bad. It's just decisions about competing claims to services. No big deal. As a concept it makes sense. However, when we look at the consequences of priority setting and the definition Klein provides for rationing, we see the truth of the situation:

> Rationing describes the effect of those [priority setting] decisions on individual patients, that is, the extent to which patients receive less than the best possible treatment as a result.
>
> *(Klein, 2010)*

Think about that for a second because the above definition is the direct result of political decisions that are made about healthcare. It means that patients get 'less than the best possible treatment' (Klein, 2010). Put more bluntly, it means that you, as their healthcare professional, give them, your patient, less than the best possible care that you could. That you are effectively withholding services (though not willingly) that could benefit your patients because of cost (Williams et al., 2012, p. 6). Tough pill to swallow as a healthcare professional—and depending on your trust's budget, you might not even be able to afford the pill.

Given it sounds nasty and counter-productive to good healthcare and good health, why do we need to 'set' priorities or ration to begin with? Well, for starters, as we've discussed above, there is normally a limited budget for state-provided healthcare. This means that by definition, there will be things that cannot be funded. In the United Kingdom, we have some more specific reasons why we need to ration within the NHS.

First, we have an ageing population with an increasing incidence of chronic diseases and public health challenges such as obesity and health inequalities. The United Kingdom is 'top heavy' with older people, meaning that more of the population needs healthcare than previous generations; they also need that healthcare for longer, as we are still (mostly) living longer than previous generations (Office for National Statistics, 2024). Medical advances are increasingly complex, as are the drugs and technology that help with treatment, and this means the healthcare system now costs more than it did in previous years. The NHS is also an incredibly comprehensive healthcare system that includes subsidised prescription medication, dentistry and physiotherapy (NHS, n.d.).

Government spending on the NHS has tried to keep up with demand, but even pumping in the huge numbers that it does, the service often doesn't manage to keep its proverbial head above water. Consider the difference in spending in the last 15 years. The NHS budget in 2010–2011 was £139.7 billion (Arnold and Jefferies, 2025). By 2024–2025, this had risen by 41%, to £197.2 billion, and yet the NHS was still unable to provide effective services (Arnold and Jefferies, 2025). In fact, even with this 41% increase in funding, the NHS is now offering fewer services than in 2010, and these figures are before we account for the actual loss in budget, as funding is not keeping up with inflation (The Health Foundation, 2024).

Types of rationing

We can understand why we need to ration, but how do we do it in practice? In healthcare, rationing largely falls into two categories: implicit rationing and explicit rationing. Implicit rationing occurs when the reason for a decision to withhold some aspect of care is not disclosed, nor is it publicly available (Scheunemann and White, 2011). Explicit rationing is the opposite, with decisions made based on explicit and defined rules of resource availability and entitlement (Scheunemann and White, 2011). Before the 1990s reforms, the NHS relied mainly on implicit rationing. Clinicians made decisions within overall budgetary constraints and patients believed care was offered (or withheld) on the basis of clinical need. While there are positives to implicit rationing— for example it allows for a more tailored approach to patients, accounting for the complexity of their problems and their preferences—it is also open to abuse. It can lead to discrimination and inequities (Mechanic, 1995). In addition, it is probably no great shock that healthcare professionals are not very comfortable making implicit rationing decisions. The NHS now uses explicit rationing for the most part. I say 'for the most part' because resource allocation using implicit rationing still exists. For example, in intensive care units (ICUs), it is not uncommon to move someone out of the unit even though they might have benefited from a couple more days of monitoring in intensive care, as they can still recover well enough out of the ICU, thus making room for someone more in need (Scheunemann and White, 2011).

Explicit rationing, where decisions are made based on known rules for resource allocation, is a way to avoid concerns with implicit rationing. It is transparent and accountable. In the United Kingdom, it is largely evidence-based, with opportunity for review and debate, thus providing more equity in decision-making (Scheunemann and White, 2011). However, like implicit rationing, there are issues with explicit rationing. It is very complex and time consuming. It can cause issues of trust and even hostility between patients and healthcare professionals. Explicit rationing also limits clinical freedom and can cause patient distress (Mechanic, 1995).

In the United Kingdom, NICE provides guidance on whether treatments (new or existing) can be recommended for use in the NHS (NICE, n.d.). NICE appraises significant new drugs and devices to 'help make sure that effective and cost-effective products are made available to patients quickly and to minimise variations in the availability of treatments' (NICE, n.d.). Once national guidance has been issued by NICE, it is supposed to replace local recommendations—the idea is that this promotes equal access for patients across the country.

However, this is not always the case. How many of you have read about the 'postcode lottery' around access to IVF treatment? It is a good example of rationing in practice, where things might look equitable on paper but are not in reality.

NICE guideline CG156 recommends that 'women under 40 years old, who have tried to get pregnant for two years of regular unprotected intercourse or 12 cycles of artificial insemination, should be offered three full cycles of IVF' (NICE, 2013 [2017]). However, in most places in England a patient can only get one cycle on the NHS; the rest have to be self-funded, and even that one NHS-funded cycle is subject to strict guidelines (Health Awareness, n.d.). I bring up this example to show how complex resource allocation decisions can be; there are national guidelines, but these are often not strictly adhered to at the local level because the service is being rationed in order to cut costs. The reason? National guidelines do not necessarily translate into national funding that supports those guidelines. There is a gap between clinical guidance and the necessary funding needed to enact that guidance. This means that individual trusts must ration certain services like IVF, and this is most often done using the economic concept of opportunity costs.

Indulge me in a brief foray into health economics.

Opportunity costs are a way of considering where to spend resources. The idea is that once you have used a resource in one way, you no longer have it to use in another way, especially if the resources are limited. In simple terms, if you have £5 and you spend it on object A, then you don't have £5 to spend on object B. The 'opportunity' to buy object B over object A is lost. Healthcare is similar. When a healthcare system decides to spend resources on a new treatment, those resources cannot now be used on other treatments because the budget is fixed. The opportunity cost of the new treatment is the value of the next best alternative use of those resources. This means that cost is viewed as a sacrifice rather than financial expenditure, and so opportunity cost is measured in benefits that are lost, not gained.

Stay with me.

Let us return to our example of IVF and examine it as a resource from a health economics point of view. The price can vary wildly, but one course of IVF costs anywhere from £5,000 upwards (HFEA, n.d.). For our purposes, we will set the price at £5,000. The recommended number of cycles is three, which would put the overall cost, if every trust followed NICE guidelines, at £15,000. To give you some perspective on this, in Canada, where I'm from, IVF is self-funded and costs between £9,000-£15,000 a cycle, putting the overall cost of three cycles at £27,000 to £45,000 (Dove, 2024). When you look at it that way, £5,000 seems to be pretty good value for money.

Now, remember that there is no guarantee that three cycles will result in a live birth. Infertility is also not a life-limiting or life-threatening condition. Some argue that it is not even a medical condition at all, but an artefact of the medicalisation of birth in the mid-twentieth century. So, all that considered, is it still good value for money?

What about if we look at some other things we can fund with the money the NHS spends on IVF? Remember, opportunity costs mean once the money is spent on one thing, it cannot be used for another. That opportunity is lost. What if I told you that £15,000 could instead fund 1,419 MMR vaccinations, half a heart bypass operation and four and a half cataract surgeries (NHS England, 2025)? Does that change how you feel about the use of the money for IVF? Is it good value for money? More importantly, is that what matters in health? You don't have to answer that question. No one should.

How do you choose?

These comparisons of resource implications and benefits of alternative ways of delivering healthcare might feel a bit like comparing apples to oranges, but it does facilitate decisions so that they are fairer and more transparent. An economic analysis compares the inputs (resources) and outputs (benefits and value attached to them) of alternative interventions. This allows better decisions to be made about the interventions that represent the best value for investment.

Now, before we go any further, I want you to think about the language that we *have* to use when we talk about healthcare economics.

Is healthcare an investment on which we need to see returns?

Are people and stock markets comparable?

Don't get me wrong. As future healthcare professionals, you need to understand how healthcare economics impacts on healthcare access, services and providers because the system you will work in will care about these things. Resource scarcity and allocation models will be in your future practice; the better you understand them, the better you can navigate them to best care for your patients. But I also want you to consider whether patients are people or numbers, or increasingly both—because it sits very uncomfortably with the way we understand person-centred care and the goal of treating each patient with dignity. Can we even measure 'cost' when it comes to health and a human life? (The answer, unfortunately, is yes, but you don't have to like it. I know I don't).

The concept of 'costs' in healthcare is incredibly complex. It goes beyond the pounds-and-pence cost of an item or service. It involves identifying, quantifying and valuing the resources needed. Resources like: healthcare services, the patient's time, caregiving costs, illness costs and the costs borne socially (such as costs to employers, families, etc. due to ill health). As Figure 6.6 shows, these are all brought together to calculate the overall cost of (ill) health. Each of these has a value and can simply be added up to identify the cost (Figure 6.6).

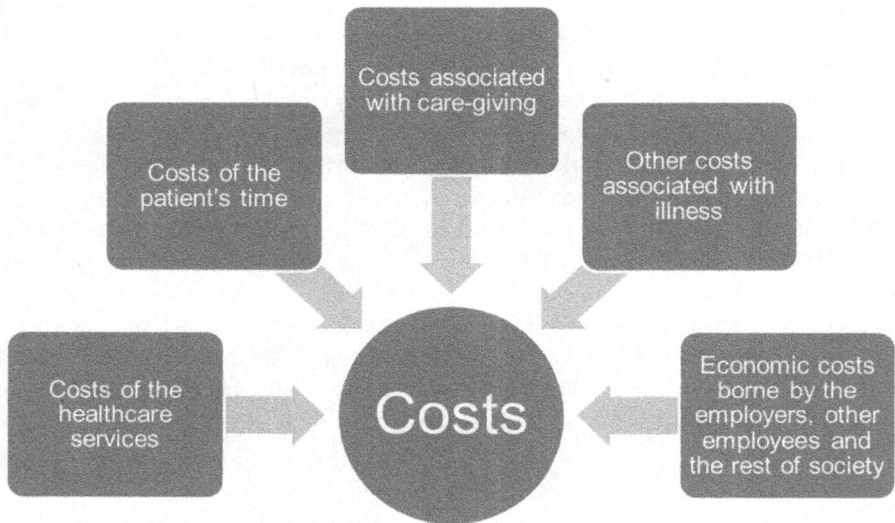

Figure 6.6 What Goes into Calculating the 'Cost' of Health.

What is much harder in healthcare is how to calculate benefit. It is almost impossible to put a value on health. Though—spoiler alert—healthcare economics gives it a good go. Mostly, benefit is considered in terms of:

1. Impact on health status. This might be in terms of survival or quality of life or both, depending on the calculations used (More on that shortly.).
2. Savings in other healthcare resources such as drugs, hospitalisations, procedures, etc., if the patient's health state is improved.
3. Improved productivity if the patient (or their family member) returns to work earlier.

Once you are able to identify these costs and benefits, you can compare them to try and find the 'thing'/resource/etc. that offers the most benefit for the least amount of cost (Williams et al., 2012). There are different ways to do this in economics, but as the NHS is our case study, we will focus on the approach that it uses, which is cost utility analysis (UK Government, 2020). Cost utility analysis is a particular type of cost effectiveness analysis. Cost effectiveness analysis is most often used to compare drugs or interventions that have a common health outcome, for example a drug that produces a reduction in blood pressure. It is very simple: different interventions or drugs are compared in terms of cost per unit outcome. With our blood pressure example, cost effectiveness analysis would look at cost per reduction of (for example) 5mm/Hg for each drug compared. This doesn't mean that the cheapest option is always chosen though. The benefit also matters. If costs are higher for one treatment, but benefits are too, then we have to calculate how much extra benefit is obtained for the extra cost. Cost effectiveness analysis asks the question: is extra benefit worth extra cost?

As a type of cost effectiveness analysis, cost utility analysis focuses specifically on quality of health outcomes produced or foregone (Williams et al., 2012). In the NHS, this is most frequently measured by quality adjusted life years (QALYs) (UK Government, 2020). Interventions can be compared in cost per QALY, and decisions to use that intervention or drug are made based on the QALY calculation.

Before we cover this calculation, I want to add a friendly reminder: QALYs are an arbitrary measurement. Like a kilo or a pound, they help to compare the value of costs and benefits in human terms. They are not a way to judge the worth of a person's life. There has been confusion over this in the past and I've been pretty vocal about how wrong it is to use QALYs in this way (Paton, 2021). Instead, what QALYs are used to work out is: if a patient takes this drug/has this intervention, how long will they be able to live their best life? It brings together quantity of life and quality of years. One year of perfect health = one QALY. This can mean a lot of things. You can trade off survival and quality of life with a QALY. For example:

1 QALY = 1 year of 100% perfect health
1 QALY = 2 years at 50% perfect health
1 QALY = 10 years at 10% perfect health

QALYs can also be used to look at more than one person. For example:

1 QALY = 12 months of healthy life for 1 person
1 QALY = 6 months of healthy life for 2 people

You can fiddle with QALYs in a number of ways, which ultimately makes the measurement a bit meaningless, but as I said above, it is more about allowing comparison than judging what constitutes a perfect life. QALYs are just a tool.

Calculating and using QALYs

The best way to understand how QALYs are used in a healthcare system is with an example.

Consider Allan. He has cancer. He is told he has one year to live if he does not have treatment for his cancer. His quality of life, without treatment, will be 0.8 (80% perfect health) and he will then die quickly. To calculate the QALYs associated with this choice we simply multiply the time frame (1 year) by the proportion of perfect health (0.8).

1 year x 0.8 perfect health = 0.8 QALY

So, choosing the option of 'no treatment' is equal to 0.8 QALYs.

If Allan receives treatment he will live for four years, but his quality of life won't be as good: it will be 0.2 (20% perfect health). Again, we multiply the time frame (four years) by the proportion of perfect health (0.2):

4 years x 0.2 perfect health = 0.8 QALYs

This means that treatment would equal 0.8 QALYs gained. In this case, between treatment and no treatment, there is no difference in QALYs associated with treatment. However, there is a big difference in terms of quality of life and length of life associated with treatment. This is why we have to be careful about how we use QALYs. Technically, comparing treatment and no treatment shows there is no change in QALYs. You can see how using QALYs to make decisions about which option to offer the patient could be used to justify not allocating resources, if the idea is that one year of almost perfect life is equal to four years of pretty crappy life. But who decides what good or bad quality of life is? Surely it's the person living it? Your patients may value one year to live to the fullest, or they may want those four years so they can reach an important goal like a 10-year anniversary or their daughter's 18th birthday. Resource allocation like this puts the healthcare professional in an awkward and morally uncomfortable position because this kind of decision is more personal than clinical. Remember, too, that the option of 'no treatment' wouldn't be cost-neutral; there would be palliative care costs involved. Both options cost money. This brings us to the next part of the overall equation: to understand fully how QALYs are used, we now need to incorporate money into the QALY calculation.

Let's use Allan again, but this time, let's be kind to him and not give him cancer.

To really understand which treatment we should use, we need more information about Allan. Allan is diagnosed at age 54 with a peptic ulcer. He can expect to live 23 years with a quality of life of 0.7 (70% perfect health) without treatment. We know how to calculate this:

23 years x 0.7 perfect health = 16.1 QALYs without treatment

There are two treatment options for Allan: Treatment A and Treatment B. They cost different amounts and produce different results, meaning different quality of life. This means we need to compare both the costs and the benefits to understand which treatment is the best value for both money and quality of life gained.

Treatment A:

Quality of life with Treatment A is 0.95 (95% perfect health) at a cost of £50 per year. Remember, Allan is predicted to have 23 years of life remaining. First, we have to calculate the QALYs associated with Treatment A:

23 years x 0.95 perfect health = 21.85 QALYs with Treatment A

Given that no treatment is equal to 16.1 QALYs, we can calculate the QALYs gained from Treatment A:

21.85 (with Treatment A)–16.1 (without treatment) = 5.75 QALYs gained from Treatment A

We also know how much Treatment A costs: £50 per year. This means we can work out the total cost of treating Allan with Treatment A for the rest of his life (predicted to be 23 years):

23 (years expected to live) X £50 (cost per annum) = £1,150 total cost of Treatment A

Finally, we can figure out exactly how much each QALY gained from Treatment A will cost by dividing the total cost of the treatment by the QALYs gained.

£1,150 ÷ 5.75 = £200

This means that each QALY gained from Treatment A costs the healthcare system £200.

Now we have to do this all over again with Treatment B.

Quality of life with Treatment B is 0.80 (80% perfect health) at a cost of £30 per year.

0.8 x 23 = 18.4 QALYs for Treatment B
18.4 (Treatment B)—16.1 (no treatment) = 2.3 QALYs gained from Treatment B
23 (years expected to live) x £30 (cost per annum) = £690 total cost of Treatment B
    £690 ÷ 2.3 = £300

This means that each QALY gained from Treatment B costs the healthcare system £300.

Treatment A is more expensive overall, but when you compare benefits and costs with QALYs, it is also more cost-effective. This means that the QALYs are ultimately cheaper because the treatment produces a better quality of life. Thus, Treatment A would be the treatment chosen by the healthcare system because it provides QALYs at a cheaper cost than Treatment B.

QALYs aren't the only measurement option out there. You may see alternatives such as Health Year Equivalents (HYEs), Saved-Young-Life Equivalents (SAVEs) and Disability Adjusted Life Years (DALYs) (Williams et al., 2012). I have focused on QALYs because the NHS, which is our case study in this chapter, follows NICE guidelines for resource allocation and NICE currently use QALYs (UK Government, 2020). As the NHS uses explicit rationing, NICE makes the rules about the drugs/interventions/technologies it will approve and decline for regular use (Bouvy, 2024).

If it is below £30,000 per QALY, the intervention/drug/resource will normally be approved as it is considered 'good' value for money. Anything over £30,000 tends to be decided on an individual case. Sometimes, people do not get the drugs that could help them the most due to cost. Enhertu, a breast cancer drug, is one of many that have hit the headlines in recent years; NICE has not approved it, as it considers that the drug is not good value for money (Burns and Loader, 2024), in part because it does not extend life for very long. The sad truth is that when there isn't an infinite pot of money, some people die earlier than they could have. That is the true result of rationing.

Understandably, there is controversy about the values embodied by QALYs. QALYs do not distribute resources according to need, but according to the benefits gained per unit of cost. Thus, all patients are treated as if they are identical, but we know they are not. We don't have a homogenous population of patients. Different areas of Britain (as we have already seen) have different resource needs. However, for the purposes of making resource allocation decisions, NICE treats all patients as if they are all exactly the same: the same background, the same access to services, the same advantages and disadvantages. QALYs also do not assess impact on carers or family, or anything beyond the medical life of the patient. In many ways, they operate in a vacuum, divorced from the environment in which the patient and the doctor live, and yet they dictate what treatments can be offered to patients and ultimately decide what is financed to maintain and improve the population's health. As the previous chapters have taught us, practising health in a vacuum, without considering the context in which people live, is a recipe for poor healthcare and increased health inequalities. Like so much of healthcare, resource allocation is not perfect. Ideally, we want a healthcare system with unlimited resources. However, that perfection is impossible to achieve, and thus things like QALYs become a necessary evil to ensure that the healthcare system remains relatively fair and functional.

Conclusion

In this chapter, I have explained how politics weaves its way into the healthcare system, as political ideology influences the political, policy and financial decisions that are made by government about the healthcare system. These change over time, and, as a result, the NHS has had to reinvent itself several times since its beginning, often with much less money and fewer resources than it had in its previous incarnation. In 2025, as I write the first edition of this book, the survival of the NHS over the next ten years remains an open question. There is little political will to embrace the kind of widespread changes needed to ensure the NHS and its complementary services, such as social care, are sufficiently funded to meet future healthcare needs. Increasingly, it is being asked to do more with significantly less, while the population it cares for continues to get bigger, live longer and be more ill than previous generations. Aspirations for better community care and integrated health and social care systems would require the government to release amounts of money from the overall budget previously unheard of in the United Kingdom's history and also to ring-fence that money for many decades to come—protecting the healthcare system from the slings and arrows of warring political parties and changing political ideologies. So far, the British government has not been able to sustain that level of commitment, and so the future of the NHS is at present uncertain and rather bleak. Don't worry. If you found that depressing, the next chapter is on climate change, so it doesn't really get any better from here. Sorry.

Test Yourself

1. You have a 42-year-old patient with breast cancer. If treated with Herceptin she will live for 17 years with a quality of life of 0.7. Without treatment she will live for four years with a quality of life of 0.3. Calculate the QALYs gained from treatment with Herceptin.

2. A new treatment for breast cancer has been developed, Senbrestat. It provides 19 years of life, but at 0.65 quality of life. It costs £23,000 per year. Herceptin costs £28,000 per year. NICE has asked you to identify which of the two treatments, Sebrestat or Herceptin, is the best overall value. Show your calculations and provide an argument for your choice.

3. Which of the four models in this chapter describes the following system of healthcare: healthcare is delivered by private healthcare providers financed by an insurance system.
   (a) Out of Pocket Model
   (b) Bismarck Model
   (c) National Health Insurance Model
   (d) Beveridge Model

4. What is an integrated care system in healthcare?

5. What kind of economic evaluation does the NHS and Department for Health and Social Care use to make decisions about what they fund?
   (a) Cost-benefit analysis
   (b) Cost minimisation analysis
   (c) Scarcity analysis
   (d) Cost utility analysis

References

Age UK (2024). *2 million older people now have some unmet need for social care.* Available at: https://www.ageuk.org.uk/latest-press/articles/2-million-older-people-now-have-some-unmet-need-for-social-care

Alsan, M., Neberai, Y. and Ye, X. (2024). 'Why the US doesn't have national health insurance: The political role of the AMA.' *Vox EU*, 9th July. Available at: https://cepr.org/voxeu/columns/why-us-doesnt-have-national-health-insurance-political-role-ama

Appleby, J., Thompson, J. and Jabbal, J. (2015). *How is the NHS performing? Quarterly monitoring report (QMR) 16.* London: The King's Fund. Available at: https://qmr.kingsfund.org.uk/2015/16/ [accessed 9th May 2025].

Arnold, S. and Jefferies, D. (2025). 'The NHS budget and how it has changed.' *The King's Fund*, 19th June. Available at: https://www.kingsfund.org.uk/insight-and-analysis/data-and-charts/nhs-budget-nutshell

BBC (2024). *Libertarianism: What is it? A simple guide.* [Video] Available at: https://www.bbc.co.uk/videos/c25lg9wxeqpo

BBC News (2011). 'Coalition government: The first 12 months.' *BBC News*, 10th May. Available at: https://www.bbc.co.uk/news/uk-politics-13062027

Bevan, G., Karanikolos, M., Exley, J., Nolte, E., Connolly, S. and Mays, N. (2014). *The four health systems of the United Kingdom: How do they compare?* The Health Foundation. Available at: www.nuffieldtrust.org.uk/sites/default/files/2017-01/4-countries-report-web-final.pdf

Beveridge, W. (1942). *Social insurance and allied services*. London: His Majesty's Stationary Office.

Boissoneault, L. (2017). 'Bismarck tried to end socialism's grip—By offering government healthcare.' *Smithsonian Magazine*, 14th July. Available at: https://www.smithsonianmag.com/history/bismarck-tried-end-socialisms-grip-offering-government-healthcare-180964064/

Bouvy, J. (2024). 'Should NICE's cost-effectiveness thresholds change?' *NICE*, 13th December. Available at: https://www.nice.org.uk/news/blogs/should-nice-s-cost-effectiveness-thresholds-change-

Burns, C. and Loader, V. (2024). 'Breast cancer patients denied life-extending drug in cost row.' *BBC News*, 18th October. Available at: https://www.bbc.co.uk/news/articles/c7v6g9q6rjqo [accessed 28th May 2025].

Clement, M. (2023). *The founding of the NHS: 75 years on*. Available at: https://history.blog.gov.uk/2023/07/13/the-founding-of-the-nhs-75-years-on/

Darzi, A. (2024). *Independent investigation of the National Health Service in England*. Available at: https://assets.publishing.service.gov.uk/media/66f42ae630536cb92748271f/Lord-Darzi-Independent-Investigation-of-the-National-Health-Service-in-England-Updated-25-September.pdf

Day, C. (2017). 'The Beveridge Report and the foundations of the welfare state.' *The National Archives*, 7th December. Available at: https://blog.nationalarchives.gov.uk/beveridge-report-foundations-welfare-state/

Doheny, S. (2015). *The organisation of the NHS in the UK: Comparing structures in the four countries*. National Assembly for Wales. Available at: https://senedd.wales/media/yqwky5az/15-020.pdf

Dove, N. (2024). 'IVF, fertility help costs are rising. For many that means "reconsidering".' *Global News*, 2nd March. Available at: https://globalnews.ca/news/10329099/fertility-costs-rising/ [accessed 12th May 2025].

Ham, C. (2023). 'The rise and decline of the NHS in England 2000–20: How political failure led to the crisis in the NHS and social care.' *The King's Fund*, 12th April. Available at: https://www.kingsfund.org.uk/insight-and-analysis/reports/rise-and-decline-nhs-in-england-2000-20

Hansard (1945). *The king's speech*. Hansard, Vol. 137, 15 August.

Harris, J. (1977). *William Beveridge: A biography*. Oxford: Oxford University Press.

Health Awareness (n.d.). *The unfair IVF postcode lottery*. Available at: https://www.healthawareness.co.uk/fertility/the-unfair-ivf-postcode-lottery/ [accessed 12th May 2025].

The Health Foundation (2024). *New analysis shows NHS budget squeezed by inflation and population growth*. Available at: https://www.health.org.uk/press-office/press-releases/new-analysis-shows-nhs-budget-squeezed-by-inflation-and-population [accessed 12th May 2025].

Hennessy, J. (2022). *A duty of care: Britain before and after COVID*. Penguin.

HFEA (n.d.). *In vitro fertilisation (IVF)*. Available at: https://www.hfea.gov.uk/treatments/explore-all-treatments/in-vitro-fertilisation-ivf/ [accessed 12th May 2025].

Kaiser, A.H., Vorn, S., Ekman, B., Ross, M., Mao, S., Koy, S., Koeut, P. and Sundewall, J. (2025). 'What contributes to out-of-pocket health expenditure in Cambodia's uncovered population? A distributional and decomposition analysis using survey data.' *Social Science & Medicine* 367: 117783. https://doi.org/10.1016/j.socscimed.2025.117783

Keisler-Starkey, K. and Bunch, L.N. (2024). 'Health insurance coverage in the United States: 2023.' *Current Population Reports (US Census Bureau)*. Available at: https://www2.census.gov/library/publications/2024/demo/p60-284.pdf

The King's Fund (2022). *Integrated care systems: How will they work under the Health and Care Act?* Available at: https://www.kingsfund.org.uk/insight-and-analysis/data-and-charts/integrated-care-systems-health-and-care-act

Klein, R. (2006). *The new politics of the NHS*. Abingdon: Radcliffe Publishing.

Klein, R. (2010). 'Rationing in the fiscal ice age.' *Health Economics, Policy and Law* 5(4): 389–396. https://doi.org/10.1017/S1744133110000095

Lambert, M. (2024). 'The vast majority of GPs resisted the founding of the NHS—here's why.' *The Conversation*, 4th April. Available at: https://theconversation.com/the-vast-majority-of-gps-resisted-the-founding-of-the-nhs-heres-why-226445

Marks, C. (2022). 'Inside the American Medical Association's fight over single-payer health care.' *The New Yorker*, 22nd February. Available at: https://www.newyorker.com/science/annals-of-medicine/the-fight-within-the-american-medical-association

Mechanic, D. (1995). 'Dilemmas in rationing health care services: The case for implicit rationing.' *British Medical Journal* 310: 1655–1659. https://doi.org/10.1136/bmj.310.6995.1655

National Audit Office (2010). *Management of NHS hospital productivity*. HC 491 (2010–11), 17th December. London: The Stationery Office. Available at: www.nao.org.uk/reports/management-of-nhs-hospital-productivity/ [accessed 9th May 2025].

NHS (n.d.). *NHS services*. Available at: https://www.nhs.uk/nhs-services/ [accessed 12th May 2025].

NHS England (2025). *2025/26 NHS payment scheme*. Available at: https://www.england.nhs.uk/publication/2025-26-nhs-payment-scheme/

NICE (2013 [2017]). *Fertility problems: Assessment and treatment*. Available at: https://www.nice.org.uk/guidance/cg156/ifp/chapter/in-vitro-fertilisation

NICE (2024). *25 years of helping to get the best care to people fast*. Available at: https://indepth.nice.org.uk/NICE-at-25/index.html

NICE (n.d.). *Making decisions using NICE guidelines*. Available at: https://www.nice.org.uk/about/what-we-do/our-programmes/nice-guidance/nice-guidelines/making-decisions-using-nice-guidelines [accessed 12th May 2025].

Office for National Statistics (2024). *National life tables—life expectancy in the UK: 2020 to 2022*. Available at: https://www.ons.gov.uk/peoplepopulationandcommunity/birthsdeaths andmarriages/lifeexpectancies/bulletins/nationallifetablesunitedkingdom/2020to2022

Paton, A. (2021). 'Jonathan Sumption has completely misunderstood what makes a life valuable.' *The Independent*, 20th January. Available at: https://www.independent.co.uk/voices/jonathan-sumption-value-of-life-bbc-big-questions-b1790014.html [accessed 28th May 2025].

Paton, A. (2022). 'I've seen the future of the NHS—with enough money, it can thrive.' *The Independent*, 3rd September. Available at: https://www.independent.co.uk/voices/how-to-heal-the-nhs-money-funding-b2158437.html

Paton, A. (2023). 'Rishi Sunak's pledge misses the real issue behind the NHS crisis.' *The Independent*, 9th January. Available at: https://www.independent.co.uk/voices/rishi-sunak-nhs-waiting-times-b2258580.html

Reid, T.R. (2010). *The healing of America: A global quest for better, cheaper, and fairer health care*. Penguin.

Scheunemann, L.P. and White, D.B. (2011). 'The ethics and reality of rationing in medicine.' *Chest* 140(6): 1625–1632. https://doi.org/10.1378/chest.11-0622

Scottish Government (n.d.). *Health and social care integration*. Available at: https://www.gov.scot/policies/social-care/health-and-social-care-integration/ [accessed 30th May 2025].

Triggle, N. (2025). 'NHS plans "unthinkable" cuts to balance books.' *BBC News*, 9th May. Available at: https://www.bbc.co.uk/news/articles/cgle2xkg3wpo

Triggle, N. and Catt, H. (2025). 'What does NHS England do? Your questions answered on health reforms.' *BBC News*, 13th March. Available at: https://www.bbc.co.uk/news/articles/crknrrz7ln6o [accessed 30th May 2025].

UK Government (1945). *Proposals for a National Health Service*. Cabinet Memorandum. CAB/129/5/39.

UK Government (2000). *The NHS plan: A plan for investment, a plan for reform.* CM 488-1. London: Department of Health. Available at: https://dera.ioe.ac.uk/id/eprint/4423/1/04055783.pdf

UK Government (2020). *Cost utility analysis: Health economic studies.* Available at: https://www.gov.uk/guidance/cost-utility-analysis-health-economic-studies [accessed 28th May 2025].

Wellings, D., Jefferies, D., Maguire, D., Appleby, J., Hemmings, N., Morris, J. and Schlepper, L. (2022). *Public satisfaction with the NHS and social care in 2021: Results from the British Social Attitudes survey.* London: The King's Fund. Available at: www.kingsfund.org.uk/publications/public-satisfactionnhs-social-care-2021

Williams, I., Robinson, S. and Dickinson, H. (2012). *Rationing in healthcare: The theory and practice of priority setting.* Bristol: The Policy Press.

CHAPTER 7

Sustainable healthcare

Future-proofing the health of Britain

The world is on fire. Sometimes literally. That the climate crisis has reached DEFCON 1 is no surprise these days. What may be a surprise, however, is that health and healthcare are wrapped up in the climate crisis—as cause, effect and possible solution. The future of health and healthcare relies as much on politics as it does on sustainability, and so in this penultimate chapter, we will look at how the healthcare of the future must be sustainable.

First, let's name the beast: climate change. The WHO has identified it as a 'fundamental threat to human health' (World Health Organisation, 2023). Climate change is a 'threat multiplier', meaning it worsens the severity of an existing or potential threat (United Nations, n.d.). Basically, climate change makes all the other awful stuff more awful. It increases the incidence of non-communicable diseases and the emergence and spread of infectious ones. It creates health emergencies through factors as terrifying as extreme weather or as workaday as reducing workforce and capacity to provide universal health coverage (World Health Organisation, 2023). There is nothing that climate change improves—it only makes things worse. And it does exist, no matter what Truth Social says.

In the United Kingdom, which has served as our case study for most of this book, climate change is viewed as such a threat to health that the GMC, the independent body in the United Kingdom that regulates doctors, physician associates and anaesthesia associates, requires future doctors to learn about climate change and practising sustainable healthcare (GMC, 2018). Sustainable healthcare is thus viewed as the future of healthcare. But I am getting ahead of myself. Before we talk solutions, first let us get to grips with the problem.

This is how the world ends (spoiler alert)

I am not going to go into the depressing details of how we got to this point. Suffice to say that it is the result of a heady mix of genuine ignorance, capitalism, globalisation, politics, greed and hubris—all of which has led to the existing crisis. The Stockholm Resilience Centre has been monitoring the situation for several decades. They identify

DOI: 10.4324/9781032677552-7

nine planetary boundaries that should not be crossed, as doing so would exceed safe limits of human pressure on the Earth (Richardson et al., 2023; Steffen et al., 2015; Rockström et al., 2009a, 2009b). Crossing these boundaries destabilises the Earth, making it less resilient to change and future pressures.

To date, as Figure 7.1 details, we have crossed six of the nine boundaries, with ocean acidification close to becoming the seventh boundary breached (Figure 7.1).

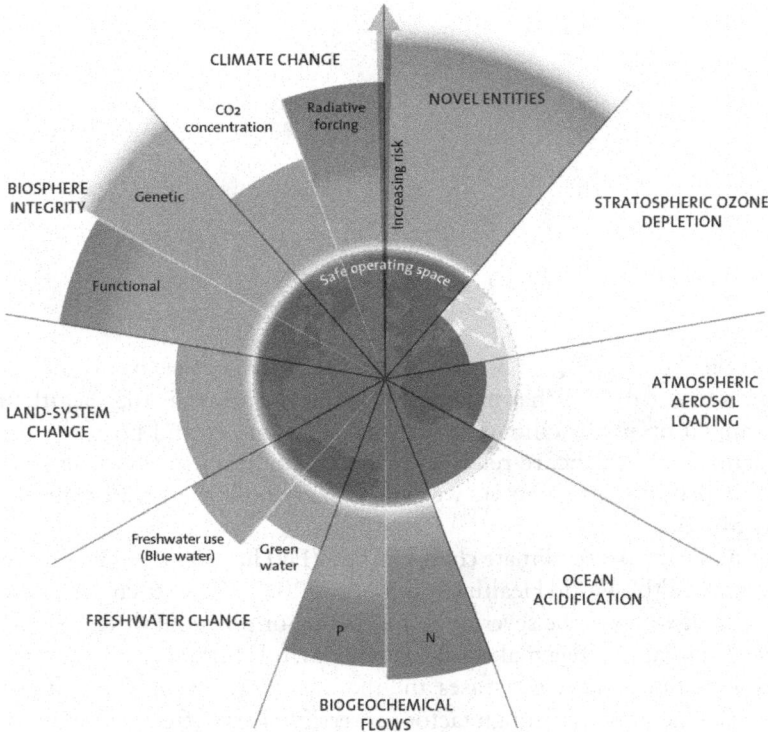

Figure 7.1 The 2023 Update to the Planetary Boundaries. Licensed under CC BY-NC-ND 3.0. Credit: 'Azote for Stockholm Resilience Centre, based on analysis in Richardson et al., 2023'

Not to be dramatic, but crossing these boundaries increases the risks of irreversible environmental change (Stockholm Resilience Centre, n.d.). Some changes will be abrupt, but many will take longer before they have an effect. The point, however, is that no matter how slow or fast the journey, we are still careening towards global environmental disaster with not much hope of stopping. These boundaries are also interconnected. They cannot be viewed in isolation, and each one that is breached puts the others at greater risk of being breached too (Stockholm Resilience Centre, n.d.). This is a long and depressing way of saying: we're in trouble.

Climate change and health

What does this mean for health? Nothing good, unfortunately. There are many different ways that climate change can impact on health. We won't cover them all in this chapter;

we'll just look at a few to give an idea of how strong this impact can be. Given that when most people think about climate change, they think about global warming, let's start there.

Global warming

Heatwaves are on the rise throughout the world due to climate change (Met Office, n.d.). Globally, a 1°C rise in temperature has occurred, causing the severity and duration of extreme heat events to increase significantly (Met Office, n.d.). The result, as we now know, is that over the last 30 years, heatwaves and extreme heat events caused by climate change have been responsible for 37% of all heat-related deaths globally (Vicedo-Cabrera et al., 2021). In fact, climate change has increased mortality on every single continent on Earth during that time period (Vicedo-Cabrera et al., 2021). In the last 25 years, the number of people experiencing a heatwave each year has increased by more than 125 million (World Health Organisation, n.d.).

The United Kingdom is of course seeing these effects. Warming is occurring in all four nations and in every month of the year (Met Office, n.d.). Extreme heat events are not only happening but also happening more frequently; they are also lasting longer. Extreme heat events in the United Kingdom have doubled or tripled in length in the last decade alone, from around five days to as many as 18 days (Met Office, n.d.). All this hot weather is not good news for health or healthcare. Hot weather worsens existing health conditions and also causes heat-specific conditions and illnesses such as dehydration and heat stroke. Heatwaves make it harder for the body to regulate its own temperature, and the strain of doing so causes an increased incidence of adverse cardiovascular outcomes such as heart arrhythmias, heart attacks and even heart failure (Mehrhof and Bunn, 2024). Organs can be strained to the point of failure, especially for those more vulnerable to dehydration. As a result, heatwaves kill, with 2,985 people dying from heat 'associated' deaths in the 2022 UK heatwave (Mehrhof and Bunn, 2024). For the over-65 age group, this number has risen dramatically, by 57% in the last 25 years, with further rises predicted (Mehrhof and Bunn, 2024). Globally, almost half a million people (485,000) die annually due to heatwaves (Johnson, 2024). Europe, in which the United Kingdom is located (despite what some MPs might say), accounts for a whopping 36% of these deaths, coming in at 175,000 per year (Johnson, 2024).

Beyond immediate impacts on the body, a warmer planet has wider health implications that may not be immediately obvious. For example, in the 2022 heatwave, IT services could not cope with the heat; three hospitals suffered IT failures as a result (Guy's and St Thomas' NHS Foundation Trust, 2023). Transport is often negatively impacted by heat, meaning people cannot access the healthcare they need when they are ill due to hot weather (Met Office, n.d.), and supply chains break down, reducing the resources available during these periods. Simple things such as ambulances are affected, with more call-outs than usual negatively effecting ambulance response time for emergencies (Thornes et al., 2014).

Air conditioning units are still relatively rare in most houses and buildings in the United Kingdom and in most NHS hospitals (except where machinery must be kept cool) (Scott, 2019). Patients swelter in ageing buildings with windows that barely open, while healthcare staff do their best to work in stifling heat. Comfort aside, extreme heat presents practical problems. I will never forget doing fieldwork in a neonatal ward during the 2018 heatwave. I watched as a frustrated and sweaty nurse was pulled from regular duty to open medicine cabinet after medicine cabinet and bin every single medication in them that could not be stored above 25°C. Waste aside, this was a logistical nightmare that then needed to be solved, as the heatwave was forecast to last for a few more days and these drugs were routinely used on the ward; they were now unavailable and restocking them risked having to bin them all again the next day. What this example shows is that extreme weather hits every part of the healthcare system hard, while simultaneously negatively impacting on the health of people in that system.

Spread of illness

Climate change is also increasing the spread of illness by increasing the risk of waterborne, foodborne and vector-borne disease (World Health Organisation, 2023). Annually, 600 million people suffer from foodborne illnesses; 30% of fatalities from these illnesses are children under 5 (World Health Organisation, 2023). Vector-borne diseases are also on the rise due to climate change. These are diseases transmitted by animals such as ticks or mosquitoes; malaria is a good example. Due to changes in temperature and humidity, more areas worldwide are becoming prone to vector growth, as they can breed more frequently in the newly warm and damp environments being created (Wellcome, 2022). Warmer climates are not only extending the transmission season of vectors, but are likely also increasing their potency, as some vectors, such as mosquitoes, tend to bite more in warmer weather (Wellcome, 2022). By 2030, it is thought that climate change will be the main reason for the expansion of vector-borne disease worldwide (Wellcome, 2022). Additionally, between now and 2070, as many as 4.7 billion people will be at increased risk to the vector-borne diseases malaria and dengue due to climate change (Colón-González et al., 2021). That's before we even get started on how climate change is likely fuelling the next pandemic, creating a perfect environment for supporting the jump of pathogens from animals to humans (Vidal, 2023). I told you this chapter would be a barrel of laughs.

Extreme weather events (or Global warming: part 2)

Climate change isn't just making parts of our world hotter; it is also creating extreme weather events that threaten our health and, in many cases, our lives. The past few years have seen an increase in forest fires, storms, flooding and drought. In the first nine months of 2024, almost a million acres of forest were destroyed by wildfire, massively impacting the health of those closest to them (European Environment Agency, 2025). This is because wildfires don't just destroy land and homes; they also cause short and long-term health problems. While the short-term issues with air quality are likely better known, let's look at the more frightening long-term impact on health caused by wildfires.

First, there is the obvious worsening of existing respiratory disease (think asthma and chronic obstructive pulmonary disease) (D'Evelyn et al., 2022). However, the impact of wildfires on health is more wide-reaching than this. Wildfires increase rates of cancer and cardiovascular disease and cause worse birth outcomes (D'Evelyn et al., 2022; Grant and Runkle, 2022). An even bigger increase in these wildfire-induced poor health outcomes has been recorded in low socio-economic groups (D'Evelyn et al., 2022). If any of you were still clinging on to the belief that health is a personal responsibility and ill health is self-inflicted, wildfires making poor people sicker has likely killed that belief stone dead.[1]

Healthcare itself, its services and infrastructure are also vulnerable to climate change. We've already seen how heat impacts on healthcare services, but other weather events are just as challenging. Flooding due to climate change, for example, is considered such an operational risk, interrupting critical services such as supply chains, energy and transport, that the NHS has started documenting these risks and how to mitigate them (NHS England, 2025). In fact, in just three years between 2021 and 2024, the number of floods recorded in NHS trusts more than doubled, from 176 to 358 (Liberal Democrats, 2024). Finally, any increase in disease due to climate change also puts incredible pressure on healthcare services and the workforce that provides those services. As future healthcare professionals, you are facing down a sweaty, waterlogged, mosquito-infested future in medicine thanks to climate change.

Climate change and healthcare: I think we might be the baddies . . .

However, as badly as healthcare is impacted by climate change, there is another, darker story here: healthcare itself is also contributing to climate change.

Six years ago, a report by Health Care Without Harm found that if the healthcare industry was a country, it would be the fifth largest emitter of greenhouse gases in the world (Bosurgi, 2019). Even with efforts worldwide to improve emissions, with a carbon footprint of 4.4% global net emissions, healthcare produces more emissions worldwide than Brazil (2.45%), international shipping (1.41%) and the whole of the United Kingdom (0.72%) (European Commission, 2024). It lags only slightly behind the European Union (6.08%) and would be the sixth largest emitter of greenhouse gases if it were a country in 2025 (European Commission, 2024). The result is that the very same entity that cares for people whose health has been impacted by climate change is also a major contributor to the problem (Bosurgi, 2019).

How has healthcare ended up in this position? Here are a few ways that it is making the problem worse. First, it has a huge beast of a supply chain, and that supply chain accounts for 71% of the emissions produced by healthcare services (Bosurgi, 2019). However, we cannot just blame other people. As Figure 7.2 shows, the way we practise healthcare, the protocols we use and the treatments needed also have a direct impact (Figure 7.2).

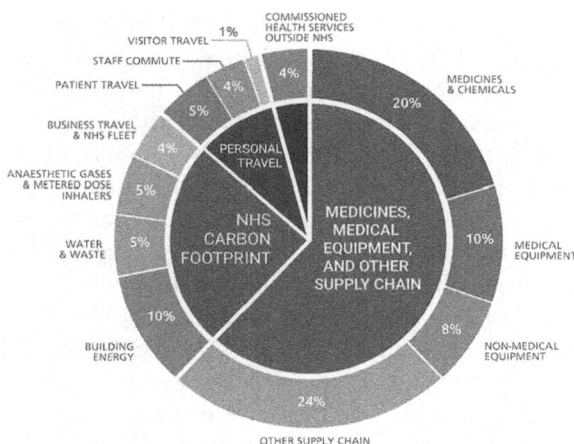

Figure 7.2 Sources of Carbon Emissions by Proportion of NHS Carbon Footprint Plus. Contains public sector information licensed under the Open Government Licence v3.0 (NHS England, 2022).

Healthcare is a big polluter. It uses all the things we aren't supposed to use: single-use plastics and aerosols. It disposes of pharmaceuticals and heavy metals and creates air pollution due to healthcare-related transport and waste disposal. It's no bastion of sustainability, that's for sure. In Europe alone, 36% of all healthcare waste is plastic waste, which cannot be recycled (Centre for Sustainable Healthcare, 2023a). Instead, it ends up in landfills or further contributes to emissions by being incinerated (Centre for Sustainable Healthcare, 2023a). This creates a vicious and health-damaging cycle whereby health waste is incinerated, releasing more CO_2 per megawatt hour than coal, gas or oil power plants, while simultaneously releasing dioxins, heavy metals and particulate matter into our air, soil and water (Centre for Sustainable Healthcare, 2023a). Once back in the cycle, these pollutants cause illnesses such as respiratory disease and cancer and damage immune and reproductive systems, leading to the use of further waste in treating those diseases and thus fuelling the cycle all over again (Centre for Sustainable Healthcare, 2023a).

Surgery is one of the worst climate offenders. For the top five most practised surgical procedures on the NHS, single-use products account for 68% of the carbon emissions produced (Centre for Sustainable Healthcare, 2023b). Worse, even reusable items still produce substantial emissions during the decontamination process—a sort of 'damned if you do, damned if you don't' worst-case scenario (Centre for Sustainable Healthcare, 2023b). Before this chapter ends the book on a low note, though, there is hope. Enter Sustainable Healthcare.

Sustainable healthcare

Many of the healthcare protocols, procedures and treatments that lead to increased emissions and pollutants have the potential to be revised in order to mitigate the impact of healthcare on the planet; this is called 'Sustainable Healthcare'. The principles of sustainable healthcare focus on reducing the carbon footprint whilst still continuing to deliver high-quality care (Mortimer, 2010). The idea is that by reducing certain activities, we reduce the impact of those activities, and in doing so provide better healthcare than before. Sustainable healthcare focuses strongly on 'upstream' healthcare, meaning things that happen before the patient even becomes a patient, such as prevention, health promotion, patient education and empowerment (Mortimer, 2010). At the same time, sustainable healthcare recognises that healthcare itself has to make wholesale changes to reach its emission goals, such as leaner service delivery, low carbon alternatives and a good awareness of its operational resource use (Mortimer, 2010). As an aside that isn't really an aside, a focus on prevention, promotion and empowerment doesn't just help the planet—it also helps tackle health inequalities in our society. Another double win.

Sustainable healthcare is under serious consideration by many healthcare systems, including our case study, the NHS. The NHS in England has committed to reaching net zero for directly controlled emissions by 2040 (what they call the NHS Carbon Footprint) and for emissions they can influence (what they call the NHS Carbon Footprint Plus) by 2045 (NHS England, 2022). They have a particularly ambitious goal of reducing emissions by 80% by 2028, which at the time of writing is only two and a half years away (NHS England, 2022). Figure 7.3 shows where all these different emissions come from. As you can see, they are varied; some are more directly under the influence of the NHS, some are not. As we already know, the supply chain is a main contributor, but the NHS currently has little control over this. In the meantime, there are other ways to engage in sustainable healthcare that can have an immediate impact. Let's return to our surgery example to see what sustainable surgery can achieve (Figure 7.3).

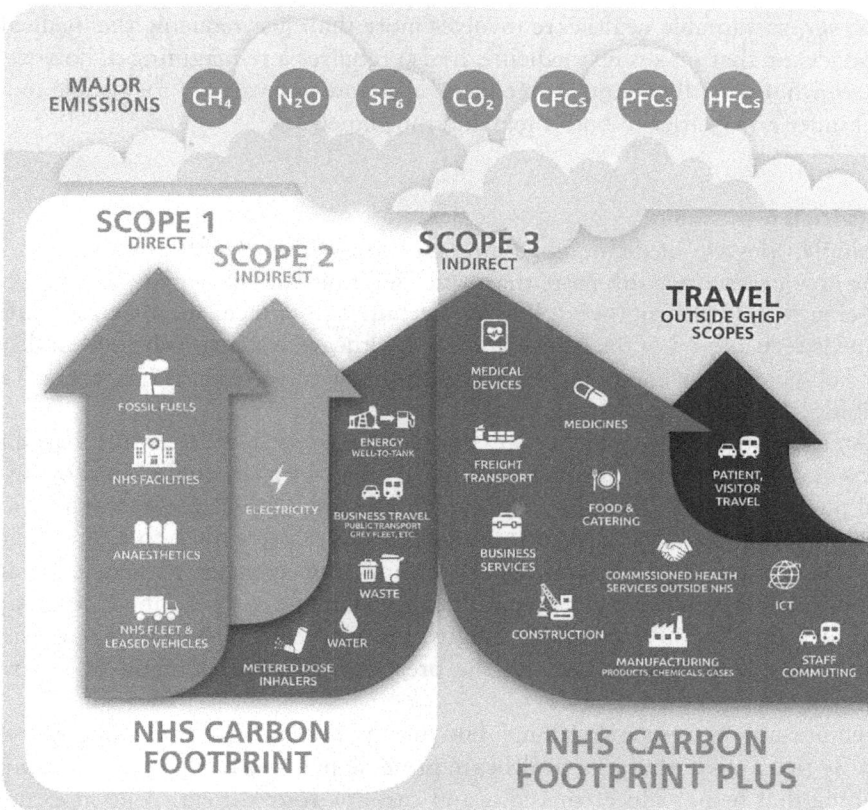

Figure 7.3 The NHS Carbon Footprint. Contains public sector information licensed under the Open Government Licence v3.0 (NHS England, 2022).

In 2021, the Green Surgery Challenge was launched. It challenged healthcare teams to propose, research and trial greener solutions to existing surgical processes that contribute to climate change (Centre for Sustainable Healthcare, 2021). The results might surprise you. They definitely surprised me. Across all five projects under study, simple changes, from asking patients to empty their bladders before surgery (to eliminate the need for catheters) to switching to reusable surgical gowns, led to better care, lower emissions and significant financial savings (Centre for Sustainable Healthcare, 2021).

Every single project saved a mid-five figure sum at minimum, between £34,000 and £88,000 per year for each procedure targeted within the project (Centre for Sustainable Healthcare, 2021). Added together across all 215 NHS trusts, this would be a whopping £19 million in savings per year that would also reduce waste and emissions—and this is just for single surgical procedures. Brought together with all the other surgery that happens in the NHS every year, this would amount to several hundred million in savings. In an era where the NHS is struggling to get by on paltry funding, a change in process that improves outcomes, reduces emissions and costs less seems like the ultimate no-brainer.[2]

However, sustainable healthcare involves more than just reducing the medical flotsam and jetsam that makes up medicine. It also requires a reimagining of how we view medicine, what actually counts as medicine and how we can care for people in a way that is kinder and gentler to both them and the planet.

Green (social) prescribing

Increasingly, lifestyle medicine is gaining traction within healthcare. With so many patients now presenting with more than one condition, and with many of those conditions being known to improve following certain non-clinical interventions, lifestyle medicine is seen as part of the future of most healthcare systems. Where lifestyle medicine and climate action combine, we can see the likely future of healthcare: green social prescribing.

Green social prescribing encourages people to engage in more nature-based interventions and activities, for example walking groups, with the goal of improving mental and physical health (NHS England, n.d.). This is a patient-centred approach that focuses on speaking to the patient to find out what matters most to them, then connecting them with the right community groups and agencies to provide practical and emotional support (NHS England, n.d.). Patients are 'prescribed' these groups through a linked member of staff, usually a social prescriber. These activities are normally considered 'green' because the prescription involves being in nature and engaging in low-carbon activities.

Green prescribing is its own 'thing', but you can regularly prescribe in a way that is 'green'. By this I mean that as a healthcare professional, you can engage in sustainable prescribing that helps reduce emissions and care for your patient. A good example is inhalers for asthma.

Most people with asthma have some sort of inhaler; the most common is a metered dose inhaler (MDI). Unfortunately, MDIs contain a powerful greenhouse gas as its propellant, often something called a chlorofluorocarbon (NICE, 2024). Chlorofluorocarbons consist of chlorine, fluorine and carbon (UK Air, n.d.). They are very stable in the troposphere, which is the closest layer of the atmosphere to Earth. This means they stay there and are subsequently broken down by the strong ultraviolet light in the stratosphere (UK Air, n.d.). During this breakdown process, chlorofluorocarbons release chlorine atoms that deplete the ozone layer (UK Air, n.d.). They are the nasty little gremlins of the greenhouse gases.

The potency of chlorofluorocarbons means that a single dose from an MDI emits as much carbon (35 kg CO_2e) as a 115-mile petrol car journey (NICE, 2024). With some

MDI inhalers having as many as 200 doses, using one is equivalent to driving the 600 miles from the north to the south of the country 38 times (NICE, 2024)! However, MDIs are not the only game in town. Dry powder inhalers can deliver the same medicine at a fraction of the carbon cost (less than 1kg of CO_2e) (NICE, 2024). This is an example where you, as a healthcare professional, can make a small but significant change that helps the climate crisis, by prescribing a greener, more sustainable medicine that still delivers quality care—thus being a prescriber who is 'green'.

Eco-distress and climate anxiety

Naturally, after such a depressing chapter, you might be feeling a little bit despondent about the future of civilisation. This is such a common response to climate change that it has not one but two names: 'eco-distress' and 'climate anxiety'. Personally, I prefer eco-distress. The word 'anxiety' can give the impression that what someone is feeling is specific to them and even 'fixable' somehow. This seems unfair given the justifiable feelings many people have in response to climate change. Eco-distress feels like a better fit. It describes the valid and understandable emotions that are felt when people learn about and engage with the impact of climate change on the planet and environment (Royal College of Psychiatrists, n.d.).

As future (or current) healthcare professionals, you may feel especially daunted, or even overwhelmed, by the contribution of your own profession to climate change. But never fear, there are ways to cope with eco-distress that don't involve solving the entire climate crisis.

First, acknowledge the distress. It sucks. We are slowly destroying our planet and, for the most part, none of us are in a position to make any major changes to stop that. Feeling upset by this is completely normal. You care about others around you—no surprise given your chosen profession. You will feel emotions about the way climate change is impacting those people. So take the time to acknowledge those emotions.

Second—and I know how cliché this sounds—small actions really do matter in combatting climate change. Think about the Green Surgery Challenge. Simple actions save millions of pounds and hundreds of tons of carbon emissions. It is that easy. If you're feeling eco-distress, take action (Royal College of Psychiatrists, n.d.). Revamp a protocol to make it greener. Plant wildflower fields. Start using a reusable water bottle at work. All of these actions count.

Third, you need to take care of yourself and your wellbeing (Royal College of Psychiatrists, n.d.). Practise self-care in whatever form that is right for you: more sleep or maybe time spent outside or with friends. Healthcare is a tough job and self-care is vital even when the world isn't burning, so take this easy 'two birds, one stone' win and find something that refuels you and makes you happy. This might mean stepping away from the news cycle about climate change, or equally it might mean engaging in the information so that you feel fully informed. Again, do what works for you.

Finally, nurture hope (Royal College of Psychiatrists, n.d.). There are more people like you out there than you think. Everywhere in the world, people are working on solutions to the climate crisis. If it helps, find those people and find out how you might further engage in what they do. Alternatively, it might simply be enough to know those people and organisations are out there. Find the balance between feeling uncomfortable enough to want to do something and comforted by the fact that so many people are doing this work. Personally, I find being the self-appointed recycling and compost Tzar of my household particularly rewarding (Note that this approach takes time as the family adjusts to saving all their apple peels and rinsing out their yogurt pots). My point is that you can change more than you think if you just give it a try—a good take-home message for this whole book, really.

Conclusion

This has been a tough chapter. It can be hard to look difficult concepts straight in the eye and understand that the very thing we do as a profession might be part of the problem. But I hope that the latter half of this chapter, with its focus on sustainable healthcare and green prescribing, has shown you that while climate change is an ever-present problem in health and healthcare, healthcare can also be part of the solution. Small actionable changes in the way you practise medicine and interact with patients will have larger, long-term rewards. As an added bonus, sustainable healthcare tends to be more equitable, cheaper and produces better health outcomes. There are upwards of 50 million healthcare professionals worldwide. If each and every one of you makes a small change, it will add up.

> **Test yourself**
>
> There are no exam questions for this section. Instead, I am setting you the challenge of identifying what aspect of your personal or professional practice that you could make 'greener'. It can be small and practical, such as using a reusable lunch box, or big and ambitious, like challenging yourself to develop a greener clinical protocol. Pick one and stick to it for a year.

Notes

1 If it hasn't, I'm really struggling to understand why you bought this book. It was a Secret Santa present, wasn't it? That's okay. It all counts towards the sales figures at the end of the day.
2 See the politics chapter to understand why this incredibly salient solution will likely not be used.

References

Bosurgi, R. (2019). 'Climate crisis: Healthcare is a major contributor, global report finds.' *British Medical Journal* 366: l5560. https://doi.org/10.1136/bmj.l5560

Centre for Sustainable Healthcare (2021). *The Green surgery challenge 2021*. Available at: https://sustainablehealthcare.org.uk/activity/green-surgery-challenge-2021/ [accessed 10th June 2025].

Centre for Sustainable Healthcare (2023a). *World Environment Day 2023: Solutions for healthcare plastic pollution*. Available at: https://sustainablehealthcare.org.uk/blog-world-environment-day-2023-solutions-healthcare-plastic-pollution/ [accessed 10th June 2025].

Centre for Sustainable Healthcare (2023b). *Single-use surgical items contribute two-thirds of the carbon footprint of products used in common operations.* Available at: https://sustainablehealthcare.org.uk/news-2023–04-single-use-surgical-items-contribute-two-thirds-carbon-footprint-products-used-common/ [accessed 10th June 2025].

Colón-González, F.J., Sewe, M.O., Tompkins, A.M., Sjödin, H., Casallas, A., Rocklöv, J., Caminade, C. and Lowe, R. (2021). 'Projecting the risk of mosquito-borne diseases in a warmer and more populated world: A multi-model, multi-scenario intercomparison modelling study.' *The Lancet Planetary Health* 5(7): e404–e414. Available at: https://www.thelancet.com/journals/lanplh/article/PIIS2542-51962100132-7/fulltext

D'Evelyn, S.M., Jung, J., Alvarado, E., Baumgartner, J., Caligiuri, P., Hagmann, R.K., Henderson, S.B., Hessburg, P.F., Hopkins, S., Kasner, E.J., Krawchuk, M.A., Krenz, J.E., Lydersen, J.M., Marlier, M.E., Masuda, Y.J., Metlen, K., Mittelstaedt, G., Prichard, S.J., Schollaert, C.L., Smith, E.B., Stevens, J.T., Tessum, C.W., Reeb-Whitaker, C., Wilkins, J.L., Wolff, N.H., Wood, L.M., Haugo, R.D. and Spector, J.T. (2022). 'Wildfire, smoke exposure, human health, and environmental justice need to be integrated into forest restoration and management.' *Current Environmental Health Reports* 9(3): 366–385. https://doi.org/10.1007/s40572-022-00355-7

European Commission (2024). *GHG emissions of all world countries.* Available at: https://edgar.jrc.ec.europa.eu/report_2024 [accessed 10th June 2025].

European Environment Agency (2025). *Extreme weather: Floods, droughts and heatwaves.* Available at: https://www.eea.europa.eu/en/topics/in-depth/extreme-weather-floods-droughts-and-heatwaves [accessed 9th June 2025].

GMC (2018). *Outcomes for graduates.* Available at: https://www.gmc-uk.org/-/media/documents/outcomes-for-graduates-2020_pdf-84622587.pdf [accessed 2nd June 2025].

Grant, E. and Runkle, J.D. (2022). 'Long-term health effects of wildfire exposure: A scoping review.' *Journal of Climate Change and Health* 6: 100110. https://doi.org/10.1016/j.joclim.2021.100110.

Guy's and St Thomas' NHS Foundation Trust (2023). *Review of the Guy's and St Thomas' IT critical incident final report from the deputy Chief Executive Officer.* Available at: https://www.guysandstthomas.nhs.uk/sites/default/files/2023-01/IT-critical-incident-review.pdf

Johnson, D. (2024). 'Heat claims more than 175,000 lives annually in Europe, latest data shows.' *UN News*, 2nd August. Available at: https://news.un.org/en/story/2024/08/1152766

Liberal Democrats (2024). *Record number of floods in NHS hospitals as trusts experience three fires a day.* Available at: https://www.libdems.org.uk/news/article/record-number-of-floods-in-nhs-hospitals-as-trusts-experience-three-fires-a-day [accessed 10th June 2025].

Mehrhof, S. and Bunn, S. (2024). 'Public health impacts of heat.' *POST*, 23rd May. UK Parliament. Available at: https://post.parliament.uk/research-briefings/post-pn-0723/

Met Office (n.d.). *UK and global extreme events—Heatwaves.* Available at: https://www.metoffice.gov.uk/research/climate/understanding-climate/uk-and-global-extreme-events-heatwaves [accessed 3rd June 2025].

Mortimer, F. (2010). 'The sustainable physician.' *Clinical Medicine* 10(2): 110–111. 10.7861/clinmedicine.10-2-110

NHS England (2022). *Delivering a 'Net Zero' NHS.* Available at: https://www.england.nhs.uk/greenernhs/a-net-zero-nhs/ [accessed 10th June 2025].

NHS England (2025). *4th Health and climate adaptation report.* Available at: https://www.england.nhs.uk/long-read/4th-health-and-climate-adaptation-report/ [accessed 10th June 2025].

NHS England (n.d.). *Green social prescribing.* Available at: https://www.england.nhs.uk/personalisedcare/social-prescribing/green-social-prescribing/ [accessed 10th June 2025].

NICE (2024). *Asthma inhalers and climate change.* Available at: https://www.nice.org.uk/guidance/ng245/resources/patient-decision-aid-on-asthma-inhalers-and-climate-change-bts-nice-sign-pdf-13558151917 [accessed 10th June 2025].

Richardson, J., Steffen, W., Lucht, W., Bendtsen, J., Cornell, S.E., Donges, J.F., Drüke, M., Fetzer, I., Bala, G., Von Bloh, W., Feulner, G. Fiedler, S., Gerten, D., Gleeson, T., Hofmann,

M., Huiskamp, W., Kummu, M., Mohan, C., Nogués-Bravo, D., Petri, S., Porkka, M., Rahmstorf, S., Schaphoff, S., Thonicke, K., Tobian, A., Virkki, V., Wang-Erlandsson, L., Weber, L. and Rockström, J. (2023). 'Earth beyond six of nine planetary boundaries.' *Science Advances* 9(37). Available at: https://www.science.org/doi/10.1126/sciadv.adh2458

Rockström, J., Steffen, W., Noone, K., Persson, Å., Chapin, F.S., III., Lambin, E.F., Lenton, T.M., Scheffer, M., Folke, C., Schellnhuber, H.J., Nykvist, B., de Wit, C.A., Hughes, T., van der Leeuw, S., Rodhe, H., Sörlin, S., Snyder, P.K., Costanza, R., Svedin, U., Falkenmark, M., Karlberg, L., Corell, R.W., Fabry, V.J., Hansen, J., Walker, B., Liverman, D., Richardson, K., Crutzen, P. and Foley, J.A. (2009a). 'A safe operating space for humanity.' *Nature* 461: 472–475. https://doi.org/10.1038/461472a

Rockström, J., Steffen, W., Noone, K., Persson, Å., Chapin, F.S., III., Lambin, E.F., Lenton, T.M., Scheffer, M., Folke, C., Schellnhuber, H.J., Nykvist, B., de Wit, C.A., Hughes, T., van der Leeuw, S., Rodhe, H., Sörlin, S., Snyder, P.K., Costanza, R., Svedin, U., Falkenmark, M., Karlberg, L., Corell, R.W., Fabry, V.J., Hansen, J., Walker, B., Liverman, D., Richardson, K., Crutzen, P. and Foley, J.A. (2009b). 'Planetary boundaries: Exploring the safe operating space for humanity.' *Ecology and Society* 14(2): 32. Available at: https://www.ecologyandsociety.org/vol14/iss2/art32/

Royal College of Psychiatrists (n.d.). *Eco distress for children and young people.* Available at: https://www.rcpsych.ac.uk/mental-health/parents-and-young-people/eco-distress-for-young-people [accessed 10th June 2025].

Scott, G. (2019). 'Why do hospitals not have air conditioning?' *Eastern Daily Press*, 26th July. Available at: https://www.edp24.co.uk/news/health/20774037.hospitals-not-air-conditioning/ [accessed 3rd June 2025].

Steffen, W., Richardson, K., Rockström, J., Cornell, S.E. Fetzer, I., Bennett, E.M., Biggs, R., Carpenter, S.R., De Vries, W., de Wit, C.A., Folke, C., Gerten, D., Heinke, J., Mace, G.M., Persson, L.M., Ramanathan, V., Reyers, B. and Sörlin, S. (2015). 'Planetary boundaries: Guiding human development on a changing planet.' *Science* 347(6223). Available at: https://www.science.org/doi/10.1126/science.1259855

Stockholm Resilience Centre (n.d.). *Planetary boundaries.* Available at: https://www.stockholmresilience.org/research/planetary-boundaries.html [accessed 2nd June 2025].

Thornes, J.E., Fisher, P.A., Rayment-Bishop, T. and Smith, C. (2014). 'Ambulance call-outs and response times in Birmingham and the impact of extreme weather and climate change.' *Emergency Medicine Journal* 31: 220–228. https://doi.org/10.1136/emermed-2012-201817

UK Air (n.d.). *What are CFCs?* Available at: https://uk-air.defra.gov.uk/air-pollution/faq?question=37 [accessed 11th June 2025].

United Nations (n.d.). *Climate change recognized as 'threat multiplier', UN Security Council debates its impact on peace.* Available at: https://www.un.org/peacebuilding/fr/news/climate-change-recognized-%E2%80%98threat-multiplier%E2%80%99-un-security-council-debates-its-impact-peace [accessed 2nd June 2025].

Vicedo-Cabrera, A.M., Scovronick, N., Sera, F., Royé, D., Schneider, R., Tobias, A., Astrom, C., Guo, Y., Honda, Y., Hondula, D.M., Abrutzky, R., Tong, S., de Sousa Zanotti Stagliorio Coelho, M., Nascimento Saldiva, P.H., Lavigne, E., Matus Correa, P., Valdes Ortega, N., Kan, H., Osorio, S., Kyselý, J., Urban, A., Orru, H., Indermitte, E., Jaakkola, J.J.K., Ryti, N., Pascal, M., Schneider, A., Katsouyanni, K., Samoli, E., Mayvaneh, F., Entezari, A., Goodman, P., Zeka, A., Michelozzi, P., de'Donato, F., Hashizume, M., Alahmad, B., Hurtado Diaz, M., De La Cruz Valencia, C., Overcenco, A., Houthuijs, D., Ameling, C., Rao, S., Di Ruscio, F., Carrasco-Escobar, G., Seposo, X., Silva, S., Madureira, J., Holobaca, I.H., Fratianni, S., Acquaotta, F., Kim, H., Lee, W., Iniguez, C., Forsberg, B., Ragettli, M.S., Guo, Y.L.L., Chen, B.Y., Li, S., Armstrong, B., Aleman, A., Zanobetti, A., Schwartz, J., Dang, T.N., Dung, D.V., Gillett, N., Haines, A., Mengel, M., Huber, V. and Gasparrini, A. (2021). 'The burden of heat-related mortality attributable to recent human-induced climate change.' *Nature Climate Change* 11: 492–500. https://doi.org/10.1038/s41558-021-01058-x

Vidal, J. (2023). 'Fevered planet: How a shifting climate is catalysing infectious disease.' *BBC Earth*, 2nd December. Available at: https://www.bbc.co.uk/future/article/20231201-fevered-planet-how-climate-change-spreads-infectious-disease [accessed 9th June 2025].

Wellcome (2022). *How climate change affects vector-borne diseases*. Available at: https://wellcome.org/news/how-climate-change-affects-vector-borne-diseases [accessed 9th June 2025].

World Health Organisation (2023). *Climate change*. Available at: https://www.who.int/news-room/fact-sheets/detail/climate-change-and-health [accessed 2nd June 2025].

World Health Organisation (n.d.). *Heatwaves*. Available at: https://www.who.int/health-topics/heatwaves#tab=tab_1 [accessed 11th June 2025].

CHAPTER 8

Conclusion

The cabbie asks me twice if this is really the address I want to go to.

'That area is no good. It's not safe.' He is adamant.

I know that. But it is also where the people who have kindly agreed to take part in my research live, so that is where I am going. As we leave the affluent area around the university and drive further towards their neighbourhood, the signs of neglect and poverty mount up. It starts with defaced bus shelters. Pretty normal, really, in most cities, but soon the defaced bus shelters turn to destroyed ones. Broken glass, missing benches and cracked windows herald a shift in the prosperity of the neighbourhood. The common green areas become less green, less frequent and more overgrown. Soon, even those show the signs of real poverty. Fly-tipped appliances and couches surround rusted playground equipment that hasn't been upgraded since the 1980s heyday of the devil-may-care approach to children's health and safety—metal slides that would burn your legs and rope bridges that could just as easily paralyse as delight sit there, dejected and frayed.

As we drive closer, my cabbie looks back at me through the rear-view mirror with greater and greater concern.

'Are you really sure, love? I wouldn't let my own daughter out here.'

I nod again. I'm sure.

When he drops me off at the house, it looks perfectly fine to me. Next door, there is a rusted-out car on blocks in the front garden. A project or a defeat, I can't tell. The front garden is surprisingly long, and as I walk towards the front door on the cracked pathway, I realise the taxi hasn't left yet. The driver is waiting for me to get inside, into what he perceives as safety.

What he doesn't know is that I do this all the time—go into houses and neighbour-hoods that for all intents and purposes reek of poverty, sometimes despair, frequently literally. When you research the world around us and the impact that it has on our

DOI: 10.4324/9781032677552-8

health, you spend a lot of time looking at poverty head-on because that's where you find the sickest people in our society. I think that tells us a lot about our world right now.

Inside might be perceived as safe by my cabbie, but it's probably more dangerous than he realises. The house is permeated by the smell of damp, rot and mould. Big black patches creep across the upper parts of the walls. The couple I've come to speak to have painted the living room a sort of purplish black to disguise its presence, but I can feel it hit the back of my throat when I breathe in.

We sit down and I'm warned to use one sofa over the other.

'The left side of that one had the bottom fall out last week!' the woman says, laughing awkwardly to hide her embarrassment.

'We bought in special biscuits!' says the man, proudly bringing out a pack of branded jammy dodgers. I take two, saying I love these (which I genuinely do), and they both beam that the expense was worth it. They want to make a good impression. They don't need to. I'm not here to judge, just to listen. I'm here to hear specifically about their experiences of caring for a pre-term baby, but while listening to that story, they give me the other pieces of the puzzle as to how they ended up living as they do.

The woman has epilepsy. She is barely able to function some days from the seizures, but the Department for Work and Pensions say she can cope on her own. It turns out she can't. She's had two seizures in the bath and has almost drowned since they started. Another occurred while holding one of her children at the top of the stairs—it could have ended in disaster. The DWP doesn't care. The boxes ticked in her assessment all indicate that she can be alone and doesn't need a carer, so she doesn't get the money for one. As a result, while she gets some meagre benefits, her partner, who has to stay home to care for her and their young children, gets nothing. The DWP deem him to be 'voluntarily' unemployed. As far as they are concerned, he has brought poverty on himself. He isn't allowed help.

'How can I go to work, knowing it could kill her?' he says at one point. Fair enough, mate. I'd stay at home too given those options.

The result is that all they can afford to rent is this damp, mouldy semi-detached in the worst area of the city. I also spot a box from the food bank in their front hall, meaning they still probably can't make ends meet. They are both depressed. Living this hand-to-mouth existence with no hope of improvement leaves them both exhausted. All five children living in the house are also exhausted. At one point their youngest, Maisy, the one born premature (but, it turns out, not the only premature baby in their family of five children), wanders in to join us. She wants a nap. She sleeps sitting up and strapped into her highchair in the living room with us, as it's the room they all find the easiest to breathe in. It has the least mould. Propped up in her chair, her lungs don't drown her in gunge. Respiratory problems are common in their house. It's so damp that it is cold on what is a hot summer's day. So much so that I'm wishing I brought a jumper.

Breathing isn't the only difficulty in this house. Half the children have some sort of neurodivergence—ADHD and autism, though the referrals are taking months, sometimes years, and the kids are struggling at school. The others have developmental delays of some sort, mostly due to being born premature. The parents are quick to tell me that neither of them smoke or drink. I believe them, not only because in my experience people are honest with me about these things but also because I genuinely don't see how they could afford a habit of any kind.

On the way out, they fall over themselves to thank me for listening to their story. They hope it helps other people have an easier time when their babies are born too soon. They are kind people. They are good people. The best I can do is to use their stories well to help the next people who come along. Maybe use it to argue for a better hospital protocol, or as evidence for the need for a change in process. But I leave feeling overwhelmed, as I often do when I spend time observing this kind of abject poverty. I don't know how to fix *this*. Fix policies that aren't fit for purpose. Fix housing associations that neglect the maintenance of their properties. Fix local authorities who are bankrupt. Fix employment that is low-paid, zero-hours and inflexible. I don't know how to fix things so that Maisy can breathe easily when she sleeps. She deserves to breathe easily. It is the most basic of human rights.

This book started with a question:

What is health?

In these chapters, we have explored just how complex this simple question really is. Health is more than our genetic disposition, inherited traits and personal choices and habits. Our world around us influences those choices, impacts on those traits and shapes our health in ways that mean we only have limited control over many aspects of our own health. We have seen how, over time, what a society or culture views as 'health' and 'healthy' changes constantly. From star signs that cure the flu to nonsensical cultural beliefs labelling sexual desire as an 'illness', we have discussed how the world we live in shapes those beliefs.

We have also seen how the true silent killers these days are the determinants of health—the way that social, structural, commercial and political forces shape health, over which most people have little control. The determinants of health are so crucial to good health that they are as important to a diagnosis as clinical symptoms. They are what keep Maisy from breathing properly in her propped-up highchair bed. They are as critical to understanding her health as the mould spores that are slowly clogging up her lungs. These determinants are responsible for the inequalities and inequities in our society that mean that people like Maisy's parents, through no fault of their own, go through life sicker than others.

Of course, regardless of where people come from, they are also individuals. Your patients will understand their health in different ways and these understandings will influence their behaviours around health. They will make decisions to safeguard their wellbeing or those of their loved ones, like Maisy's father staying home to keep his wife alive. They will be more or less able to adhere to a treatment. They will be more or less inclined to take lifestyle advice. This book has given you some tools to support your patients to make positive behaviour changes for their health—but remember, they are only tools. Trust is the key in supporting your patients. Trust in each other, but also trust in the experiences of your patient and their own expertise in themselves.

All of this said, there are some things none of us can really control, even in health. I hope that this book has helped you understand the wider context of medicine and healthcare. Just as your patients do not live in a vacuum, you will not practice medicine in a vacuum. You might be able to prescribe Maisy an inhaler or change her mother's epilepsy medication, but you will struggle to change the policies that mean they have no choice but to live in the poverty they do. Your ability to be the best healthcare professional you can and want to be will not be fully in your control. You will be helped or hampered by the political whims of the government that oversees your healthcare system. You will be supported or constrained by that healthcare system itself. Almost none of it will be consistent or predictable. And, of course, as the penultimate chapter has shown, you will be doing so while climate change irrevocably alters the world. In short, you are subject to as many societal, cultural, political, economic and environmental whims as your patients.

I hope another important realisation has occurred in the reading of this book: that, as a healthcare professional, you will mean something different to every patient you see. To some, you will be the fount of all clinical knowledge, and to others, a barrier to their own life goals. To many, you will be hope—hope that you can heal, support and understand them. To do so, you will need to use everything you have learnt from this book, combine it with your clinical knowledge and, then, as I think you understand now, remember that every patient is unique and cannot be treated the same as the patient who came before or the patient who comes next.

I'm outside their house now. I take out my phone to call for another taxi, thinking I will lounge at their gate in the sun and write my notes while I wait for my ride. A horn beeps. It's my cabbie from two hours ago. He never left, convinced I had insanely placed myself in mortal danger and determined to get me home safe in spite of myself.

'You didn't have to wait. I'm safe,' I say as I get in.

He shakes his head. 'A good person would wait,' he tells me as he drives off, still finding me inexplicably reckless.

'They're good people too,' I say in response. And they are. Every single person I meet in this job is a good person trying, but sometimes failing, through mostly no fault of their own, to make the best out of what is often an incredibly bleak situation. When they come to you sick, seeking support, wanting to trust—remember what you have learnt in this book and use it to be the healthcare professional they really need. Listen to them. Understand them. Care for them when society can't or won't. I think we both know now that you can, and you will.

Good luck.

CHAPTER 9

Test yourself

To help you with revision, should you be using this book for your studies, this section contains opportunities to test your knowledge on what you have learned. These have been written in the style of examination questions most commonly used in healthcare professional degrees, so that you can use them as a way to study. They are a mix of all the topics covered in the book, so that you can get used to the way questions may appear in your examinations. Answers are available at the end of this section, along with the answers to the Test Yourself sections at the end of each chapter.

Test 1:

Question 1.1: Identify the main difference between the behavioural-cultural and the materialist explanations.

Question 2.1: Doreen has put off going to her doctor to talk about her coughing. When Doreen finally does go see her doctor, it turns out she has undiagnosed asthma. She is shocked. She has always been a bit 'chesty' but nothing that bothered her. She doesn't like her inhaler and only uses it when she thinks her asthma is really bad. What category of health belief does Doreen's behaviour fall into?
(a) Distancer
(b) Denier
(c) Acceptor
(d) Pragmatist

Question 3.1: What are the five different aspects of the Health Belief Model necessary to modify behaviour?

Question 4.1: A new treatment for breast cancer has been developed, Senbrestat. It provides 19 years of life, but at 0.65 quality of life. It costs £23,000 per year. Herceptin, costs £28,000 per year. NICE has asked you to identify which of the two treatments,

DOI: 10.4324/9781032677552-9

Sebrestat or Herceptin, is the best overall value. Show your calculations and provide an argument for your choice.

Question 5.1: Provide a definition for the Commercial Determinants of Health.

Question 6.1: Identify and describe two limitations of Parson's 'Sick Role' concept.

Question 7: Pavlov discovered which theory of behaviour. Provide the name of the theory and a brief definition.

Question 8.1: What are the two key components of reflective listening?
(a) Talking and Listening
(b) Interrupting and Nodding
(c) Mirroring and Paraphrasing
(d) Understanding and Empathy

Question 9.1: What is sustainable healthcare?

Question 10.1: What is the WHO definition of health?

Test 2:

Question 1.2: A 7-year-old child is diagnosed with asthma. He lives in a deprived area of Birmingham where air pollution is high and the quality of housing is poor.

This relationship between socio-economic status and health is referred to as?
(a) Bad luck
(b) Health inequalities
(c) Socialism
(d) Social selection

Question 2.2: Doreen has had a cough for two weeks and is wondering whether she should go see her doctor about it. She speaks to her husband, sister and a co-worker, who all had the same cold, about how long they were ill. They all tell her it took three weeks to get better and so Doreen decides not to go see her doctor about her cough. In doing so, what behaviour has Doreen engaged in to make a decision about her health?

Question 3.2: What are the three foci of the WHO definition of health?

Question 4.2: Define health-related behaviours.

Question 5.2: How does Operant Conditioning modify behaviour?
(a) It modifies behaviour through reinforcement in the form of punishment or reward.
(b) It modifies behaviour through positive association techniques.
(c) It modifies behaviour through medication and counselling.
(d) It modifies behaviour through negative association techniques.

Question 6.2: Define 'Concordance'.

Question 7.2: What are the four levels of prevention?

Question 8.2: You have a 42-year-old patient with breast cancer. If treated with Herceptin she will live for 17 years with a quality of life 0.7. Without treatment she will live for 4 years with a quality of life of 0.3.

Calculate the QALYs gained from treatment with Herceptin.

Question 9.2: What kind of economic evaluation does the NHS and Department for Health and Social Care use to make decisions about what they fund?
(e)   Cost-benefit analysis
(f)   Cost minimisation analysis
(g)   Scarcity analysis
(h)   Cost utility analysis

Question 10.2: What is green prescribing? Give one example of green prescribing in your answer.

Test 3:

Question 1.3: Define lay epidemiology.

Question 2.3: How does the inverse care law negatively affect health?

Question 3.3: Health-related behaviours that promote good health are known as:
(a)   Good habits
(b)   Positive health-protective behaviours
(c)   Low-risk behaviours
(d)   Health promotion

Question 4.3: Biographical disruption identifies three ways that the onset of illness changes how we understand ourselves. What are these three ways?

Question 5.3: Pavlov discovered which theory of behaviour. Provide the name of the theory and a brief definition.

Question 6.3: What is the focus of population and public health?

Question 7.3: Which of the four models in this chapter describes the following system of healthcare: Healthcare is delivered by private healthcare providers financed by an insurance system.
(e)   Out of Pocket Model
(f)   Bismarck Model
(g)   National Health Insurance Model
(h)   Beveridge Model

Question 8.3: Health Promotion aims to:
(a)   Cure disease once it has reached an advanced stage
(b)   Raise education and awareness about health, disease and illness
(c)   Detect and treat disease or risk factors at an early stage
(d)   Detect who needs palliative care

Question 9.3: What is an integrated care system in healthcare?
Question 10.3: Name one way that climate change is impacting on health.

Answers

Test 1

1.1: Main difference is that the former assumes people have choice while the latter recognises that differential access to material resources can seriously limit choice.

2.1: (d) Pragmatist

3.1:
1. Perceived susceptibility
2. Perceived severity
3. Perceived benefits
4. Perceived barriers
5. Self-efficacy

4.1:
Herceptin costs £28,000 x 17= £476,000
£476,000 ÷ 10.7 = £44,485.98 per QALY gained
19 years x 0.65 QoL = 12.35
QALYs gained: 12.35–1.2 = 11.15 QALYs gained
Senbrestat costs £23,000 x 19 = £437,000
£437,000 ÷ 11.15 = £39,192.82 per QALY gained
On balance, the best option is likely Senbrestat, which costs less, keeps patients alive longer and has only marginally lower quality of life associated with it. However, it could also be argued that while it is more expensive, Herceptin provides better quality of life, and thus is worth paying that little bit extra

5.1: Commercial determinants of health are those activities in the private sector, that is areas and industries that make money, which directly and indirectly influence health in positive and negative ways.

6.1: (Accept any combination of two from the list below)
a. Not all illnesses are temporary.
b. It does not account for structural limits to a person's ability to 'be' sick.
c. It does not acknowledge differences between people, cultures or societies.
d. It does not acknowledge individual agency in defining and coping with illness.

7.1: Classic conditioning, where a new behaviour is learnt through the process of association.

8.1: (c)

9.1: Sustainable healthcare focus on reducing carbon footprint whilst still continuing to deliver high quality care.

10.1: Health is a state of complete physical, mental and social wellbeing and not merely the absence of disease or infirmity.

Test 2

1.2: (b) Health inequalities

2.2: The lay referral system.

3.2: Physical, mental and social wellbeing.

4.2: Health-related behaviour is any behaviour that has a consequence on health and/or illness.

5.2: (a)

6.2: Concordance occurs when a patient and healthcare professional agree together on the best treatment plan for the patient

7.2: Primordial, Primary, Secondary and Tertiary

8.2:

With Herceptin the patient will have 11.9 QALYs
(17 years x 0.7 QoL)
Without Herceptin the patient will have 1.2 QALYs
(4 years x 0.3 QoL)
The number of QALYs gained is 10.7.

9.2: (d)

10.2: Green prescribing is prescribing nature-based interventions and activities, for example a walking group, with the goal of improving mental and physical health for patients.

Test 3

1.3: Lay epidemiology is how a person understands why and how illness happens, and why it happened to a particular person at a particular time.

2.3: The inverse care law negatively affects health because it means that those communities that most need access to healthcare normally have the hardest time getting that access, thus they have a harder time receiving the healthcare they need to be healthier.

3.3: (b)

4.3:

(a) Disruptions of everyday activities
(b) A rethinking of self
(c) Mobilisation of resources

5.3: Classic conditioning, where a new behaviour is learnt through the process of association.

6.3: Population and public health are concerned with the overall health of groups, communities and populations.

7.3: (b)

8.3: (b)

9.3: ICSs are partnerships that bring together providers and commissioners of NHS services with local authorities and other local partners to plan, co-ordinate and commission health and care services all within one geographic area.

10.3: (not an exhaustive list):

—increases extreme weather
—increases heat events and heat waves
—increases vector-borne disease
—increases water-borne disease
—increases food-borne disease
—causes stress on existing conditions and illnesses

Chapter 2 Answers:

1. The Main difference is that the former assumes people have choice while the latter recognises that differential access to material resources can seriously limit choice.

2. (b) Health inequalities

3. Commercial determinants of health are those activities in the private sector, i.e. areas and industries that make money, which directly and indirectly influence health in positive and negative ways.

4. The inverse care law negatively affects health because it means that those communities that most need access to healthcare normally have the hardest time getting that access, thus they have a harder time receiving the healthcare they need to be healthier.

5. Health is a state of complete physical, mental and social well-being and not merely the absence of disease or infirmity.

Chapter 3 Answers:

1. Lay epidemiology is how a person understands why and how illness happens, and why it happened to a particular person at a particular time.

2. The lay referral system.

3. (d) Pragmatist

4. (Accept any combination of two from the list below)
   a. Not all illnesses are temporary.
   b. It does not account for structural limits to a person's ability to 'be' sick.
   c. It does not acknowledge differences between people, cultures or societies.
   d. It does not acknowledge individual agency in defining and coping with illness.

5. (a) Disruptions of everyday activities.
   (b) A rethinking of self.
   (c) Mobilisation of resources.

Chapter 4 Answers:

1. Health-related behaviour is any behaviour that has a consequence on health and/or illness.

2. (b)

3. Classic conditioning, where a new behaviour is learnt through the process of association.

4. (a)

5. (a) Perceived susceptibility
   (b) Perceived severity
   (c) Perceived benefits
   (d) Perceived barriers
   (e) Self-efficacy

Chapter 5 Answers:

1. Concordance occurs when a patient and healthcare professional agree together on the best treatment plan for the patient.

2. (c)

3. Population and public health are concerned with the overall health of groups, communities and populations.

4. Primordial, Primary, Secondary and Tertiary
5. (b)

Chapter 6 Answers:
1. With Herceptin the patient will have 11.9 QALYs (17 years × 0.7 QoL)
   Without Herceptin the patient will have 1.2 QALYs (4 years × 0.3 QoL)
   The number of QALYs gained is 10.7
2. Herceptin costs £28,000 × 17= £476,000
   £476,000 ÷ 10.7 = £44,485.98 per QALY gained
   19 years × 0.65 QoL = 12.35
   QALYs gained: 12.35-1.2 = 11.
   15 QALYs gained
   Senbrestat costs £23,000 × 19 = £437,000
   £437,000 ÷ 11.15 = £39,192.82 per QALY gained
   On balance the best option is likely Senbrestat, which costs less, keeps patients alive longer and has only marginally lower quality of life associated with it. However it could also be argued that while it is more expensive, Herceptin provides better quality of life, and thus is worth paying that little bit extra.
3. (b)
4. ICSs are partnerships that bring together providers and commissioners of NHS services with local authorities and other local partners to plan, co-ordinate and commission health and care services all within one geographic area.
5. (d)

Index

Note: Page numbers in *italics* indicate a figure, and page numbers in **bold** indicate a table on the corresponding page. Page numbers followed by 'n' with numbers refer to notes.

For Product Safety Concerns and Information please contact our EU
representative GPSR@taylorandfrancis.com
Taylor & Francis Verlag GmbH, Kaufingerstraße 24, 80331 München, Germany

www.ingramcontent.com/pod-product-compliance
Lightning Source LLC
Chambersburg PA
CBHW081107220326
41598CB00038B/7265